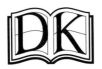

try it!

NAIL ART

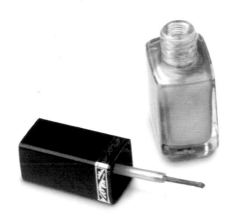

by Emily Draher

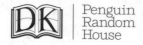

DK INDIA
Project Editor Arani Sinha
Senior Art Editor Ivy Roy
Art Editor Jomin Johny
Deputy Managing Editor Bushra Ahmed
Managing Art Editor Navidita Thapa
Pre-Production Manager Sunil Sharma
DTP Designers Nityanand Kumar and
Manish Chandra Upreti

DK UK
Project Editor Kathryn Meeker
Senior Art Editor Anne Fisher
Anglicizer Constance Novis
Managing Editor Stephanie Farrow
Managing Art Editor Christine Keilty
Jacket Designer Amy Keast
Producer, Pre-Production Andy Hilliard
Producer Stephanie McConnell

First published in Great Britain in 2016 by
Dorling Kindersley Limited,
80 Strand, London WC2R ORL

Copyright © 2016 Dorling Kindersley Limited
A Penguin Random House Company
15 16 17 18 19 10 9 8 7 6 5 4 3 2 1
001 – 286851– Jan/2016

A CIP catalogue record for this book
is available from the British Library.
ISBN 978-0-2412-2952-1

Printed and bound in China.

All images © Dorling Kindersley Limited
For further information see: www.dkimages.com

A WORLD OF IDEAS:
SEE ALL THERE IS TO KNOW

www.dk.com

Contents

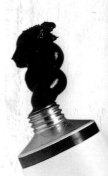

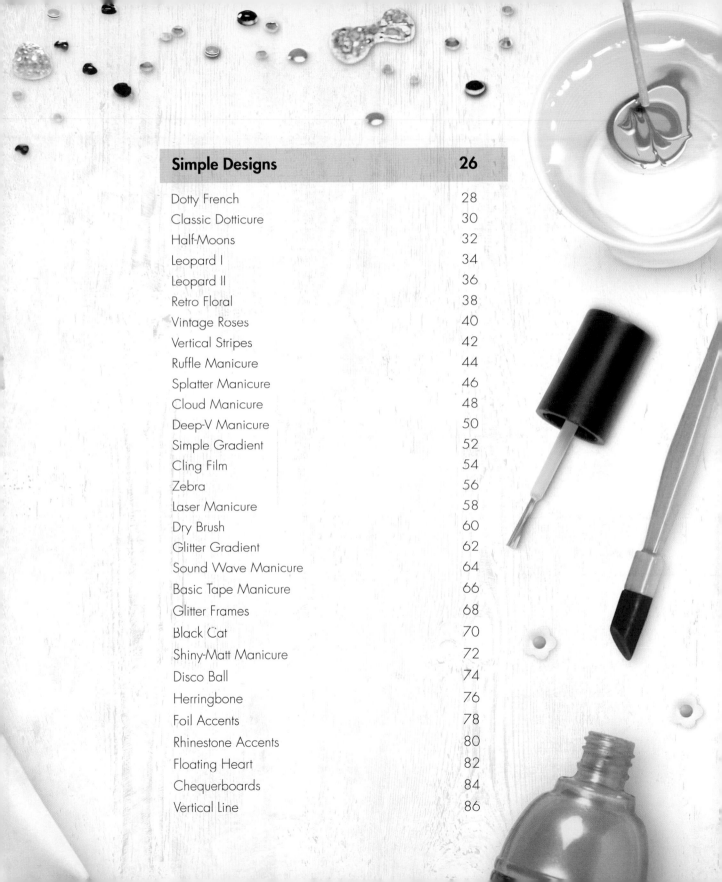

Simple Designs   26

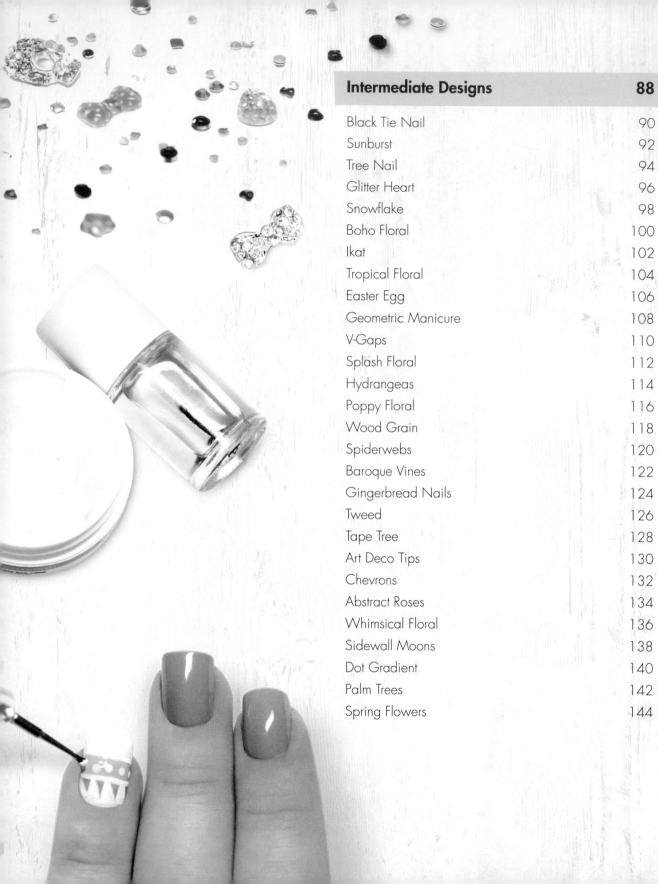

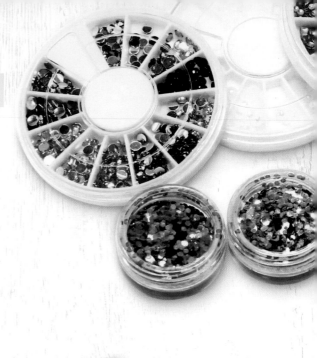

Advanced Designs 146

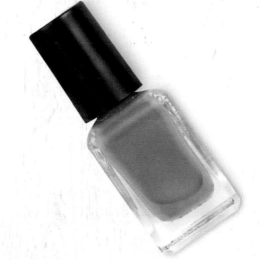

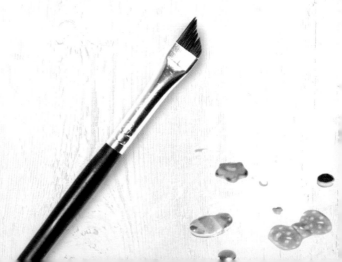

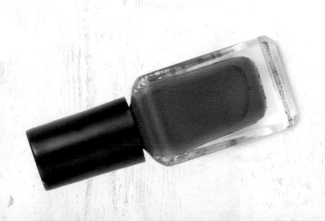

Introduction

In today's fast-paced world, no detail goes unnoticed. That's why women and girls alike are slowing down to do their own nails in striking and original ways. Your manicure is the finishing touch to your outfit, and there are no longer rules when it comes to colours or design. Nail art has taken the world by storm as a new way to express yourself: every style, personality, and mood can be communicated through colour and art. Bold colours, graphic designs, and themed manicures are available at most nail salons today, but you can also create them on yourself and your friends at home.

Colourful manicures have been part of the world of fashion for decades. While the traditional colours and looks, such as shiny red, frosty pink, and French tips are still options, it is now appropriate to wear bold colours and graphic designs on your nails. Start simply by wearing a metallic accent nail in a shade to match your accessories. Wear bright floral nails to celebrate spring, or snowflakes during the first blizzard of the season. Wear earthy, nature-inspired designs while camping or a dazzling glitter gradient for a formal black-tie affair. Try Jack-o'-Lanterns for Hallowe'en, hearts for Valentine's Day, eggs for Easter, and trees for Christmas. No matter the season or event, there is nail art that is eye-catching and appropriate for nearly any occasion.

Manicures, pedicures, and nail art are a great way to treat yourself during a stolen moment of calm, but they can also be something fun to share with the special women in your life. Almost every woman, no matter her age or style, can appreciate pampering herself and enjoy a DIY manicure. Sisters and friends can practise their nail art skills on each other, and mums and daughters can spend quality time together over a bottle of polish. Nail parties make for great birthday parties or hen nights.

This book outlines everything you need to know to explore the world of DIY nail art, starting with nail care, proper tools for manicuring and nail art, and helpful tips and tricks in Part 1. If your nails aren't in perfect shape, you can adopt proper manicuring technique and some simple daily habits, and you will see a difference in your nails within a few weeks. Many people struggle to understand how designs can be created on such a small canvas as a finger nail, but with the right tools, it can be easy. Before you get started, head to your local beauty supply shop or order the basic tools online. Other nail services you can do for yourself or your friends at home, such as soak-off gel manicures and pedicures, are discussed in Part 1 as well.

The majority of this book features tutorials for a wide variety of nail art designs, ranging in difficulty from basic to advanced. In the simple designs in Part 2, you will learn to use some of the most important nail art tools: the dotting tool, striping brush, and striping tape, as well as a variety of items from around your home. Many of the designs in this section would be appropriate to try with younger girls who are eager to do their own nails. The intermediate and advanced designs in Parts 3 and 4 combine the basics with more intricate, freehand nail art. These tutorials take you step by step through the designs, so you will not be overwhelmed. If you are just beginning, start with a simple technique and be creative. You can ring the changes by incorporating different colours and polish finishes. Keep practising the simple designs until you are comfortable with your technique, and then move on to the more difficult designs. You'll be surprised at what you are capable of just by following the tutorials in this book.

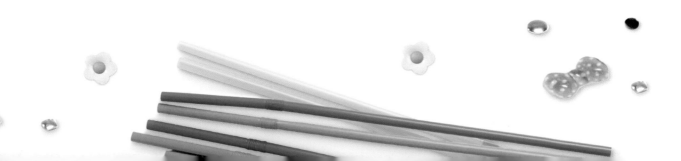

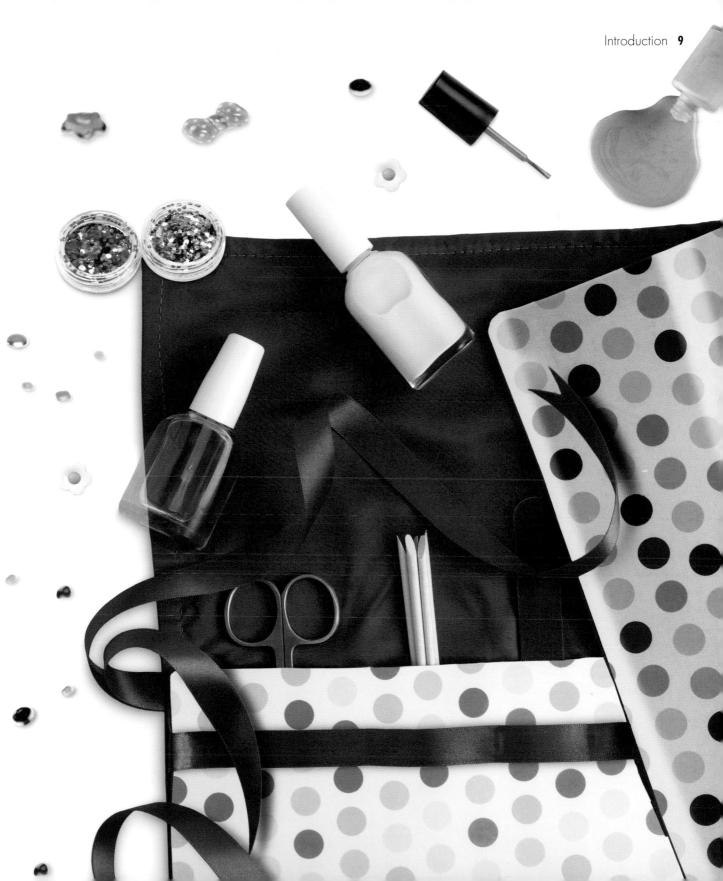

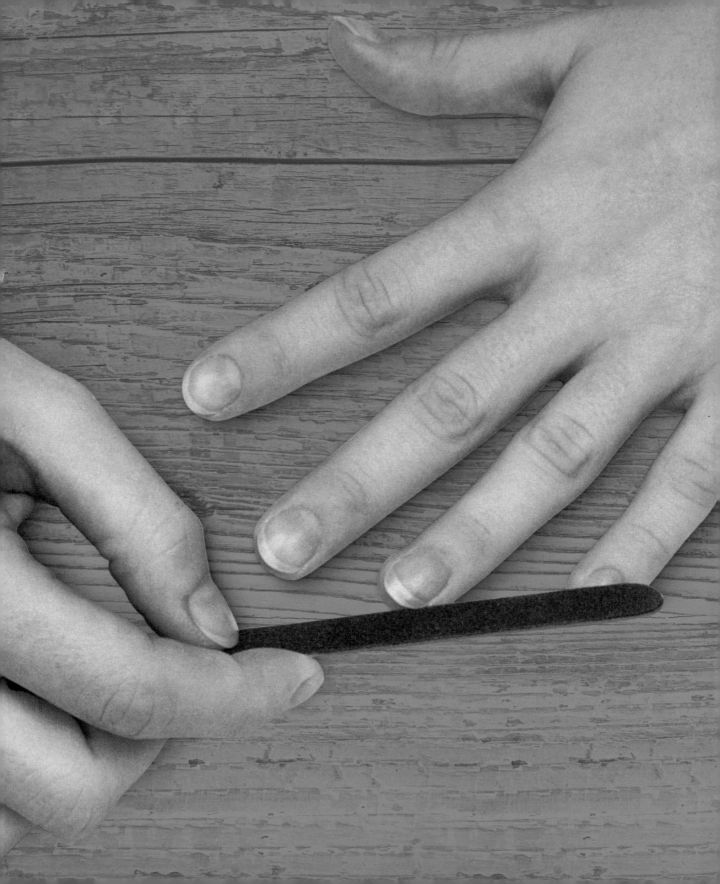

Nail Art
Basics

Before diving into the world of nail art, it's helpful to know how to take care of your nails and hands. In this section, you will learn some essential nail care basics that turn your nails into beautiful nail art canvases. Performing a DIY manicure and polishing your nails is much more rewarding when you follow a technique that produces the best results. By using a base coat, top coat, and clean-up brush, your manicures will be clean and long-lasting. You'll also learn about other polishing options, such as soak-off gel manicures, pedicures, and toenail art.

Know Your Nails

Before you can have strong, healthy nails worthy of nail art, you need to understand the basic structure of your nails so you can properly care for them. The **nail plate** is the hard part of the nail that is polished. Many people probably don't think about their nails in much more detail than the nail plate, but healthy nails begin in the **nail matrix,** which is where the living, growing cells of your nails are formed. The matrix is located under your skin at the base of your nail, and sometimes can be seen showing through under the nail plate as the **lanula,** the white half-moon shape you may see at the root of each nail.

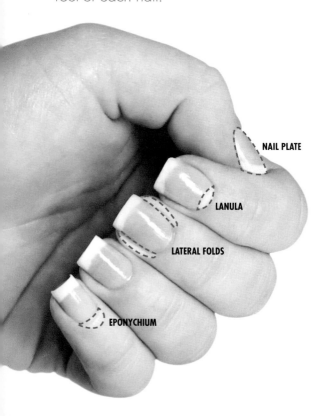

NAIL PLATE

LANULA

LATERAL FOLDS

EPONYCHIUM

STRUCTURE OF THE NAIL

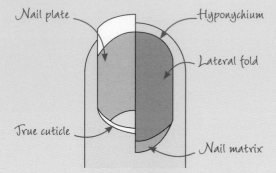

Nail plate

Hyponychium

Lateral fold

True cuticle

Nail matrix

PARTS OF A HEALTHY NAIL

In the matrix area, new nail cells are formed and pushed forwards to become part of the nail plate. If your nail matrix is healthy, your nail will grow normally. The shape of your nail matrix determines how your nails grow, which means the shape of your natural nail plate cannot be changed. If your nail matrix is harmed through trauma or infection, the nail plate can be permanently damaged.

To protect the nail matrix and prevent the entry of bacteria and other germs, the skin around your nails (the sidewall) folds tightly against the nail to create a seal. The hyponychium, under the free edge, creates a seal between the nail bed and nail plate. The eponychium is the living tissue at the base of your nail that creates a seal with the nail plate, and is often referred to as the cuticle. This is incorrect because the cuticle is the dead, sticky tissue that grows up onto your nail plate. The cuticle can be nipped and removed, but you should never cut your eponychium.

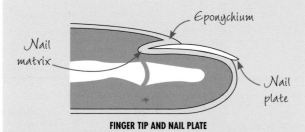

Eponychium

Nail matrix

Nail plate

FINGER TIP AND NAIL PLATE

The nail plate is made up of about 100 layers of nail cells and keratin connected together by cross-links, which help create its rigid structure. Small channels between the keratin layers usually contain water and oil. Limiting overexposure to water and using cuticle oils can help maintain moisture levels for strong, healthy nails.

Good nail habits

Regular manicures are very important for keeping your nails beautiful, but if you neglect your hands and nails between manicures, you will not see long-term improvement in their appearance and health. Here are a few simple daily habits that can make a big difference.

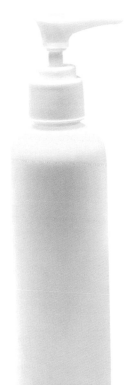

PROTECT YOUR HANDS

Exposure to water and chemicals can damage your nails and also cause your manicure to chip and look dull. If you can, avoid soaking your nails for long periods while bathing and swimming, and wear rubber gloves while doing the washing up, cleaning, or handling household chemicals. This will not only protect your nails, but will also help keep your skin away from potentially harmful chemicals and detergents.

DAILY MAINTENANCE

Daily nail maintenance is a simple way to keep your nails in shape between manicures. When you apply hand cream, take a few extra seconds to massage it into your eponychium and apply cuticle oil or cream at least once each day. Keeping your nails well oiled helps maintain a healthy moisture balance, which leads to more flexible, chip- and tear-resistant nail plates. Cuticle oils and creams can also encourage healthy nail growth and extend the life of your manicure.

   When performing your manicure at home, there are some other habits to keep in mind. Rough filing in a sawing motion can shear apart layers of your nail, leading to peeling. Always file your nails from the outside corners to the centre of the free edge, in one direction at a time. Also, when dealing with your cuticles and eponychium, be extremely cautious. The eponychium should not be cut or pushed back with force, as this can lead to nail matrix damage.

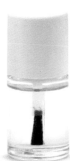

Do

Apply cuticle oil daily
Keep hands moisturized
Wear rubber gloves
File in one direction
at a time

Don't

Soak excessively in water
Expose your nails to chemicals
File with a sawing motion
Use your nails as tools
Buff excessively
Cut the eponychium

Manicure and Polish Set

To maintain healthy and beautiful nails, you need to perform regular manicures and do some daily maintenance using the products shown here.

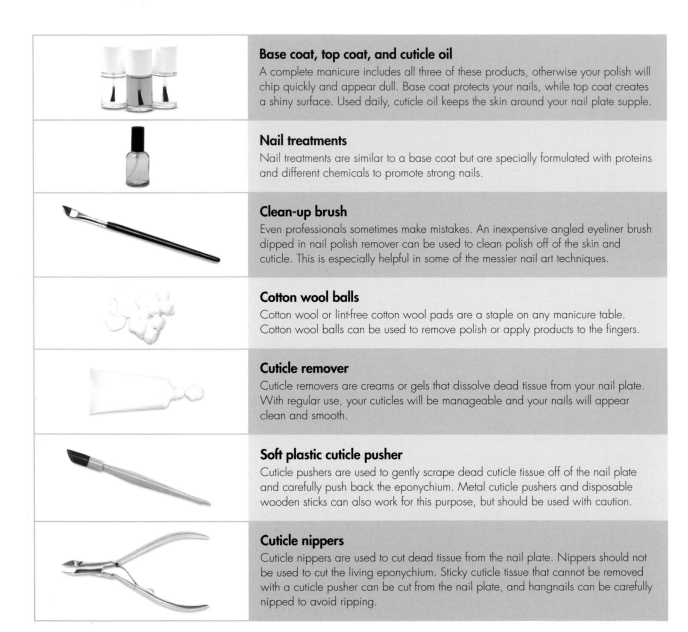

Base coat, top coat, and cuticle oil

A complete manicure includes all three of these products, otherwise your polish will chip quickly and appear dull. Base coat protects your nails, while top coat creates a shiny surface. Used daily, cuticle oil keeps the skin around your nail plate supple.

Nail treatments

Nail treatments are similar to a base coat but are specially formulated with proteins and different chemicals to promote strong nails.

Clean-up brush

Even professionals sometimes make mistakes. An inexpensive angled eyeliner brush dipped in nail polish remover can be used to clean polish off of the skin and cuticle. This is especially helpful in some of the messier nail art techniques.

Cotton wool balls

Cotton wool or lint-free cotton wool pads are a staple on any manicure table. Cotton wool balls can be used to remove polish or apply products to the fingers.

Cuticle remover

Cuticle removers are creams or gels that dissolve dead tissue from your nail plate. With regular use, your cuticles will be manageable and your nails will appear clean and smooth.

Soft plastic cuticle pusher

Cuticle pushers are used to gently scrape dead cuticle tissue off of the nail plate and carefully push back the eponychium. Metal cuticle pushers and disposable wooden sticks can also work for this purpose, but should be used with caution.

Cuticle nippers

Cuticle nippers are used to cut dead tissue from the nail plate. Nippers should not be used to cut the living eponychium. Sticky cuticle tissue that cannot be removed with a cuticle pusher can be cut from the nail plate, and hangnails can be carefully nipped to avoid ripping.

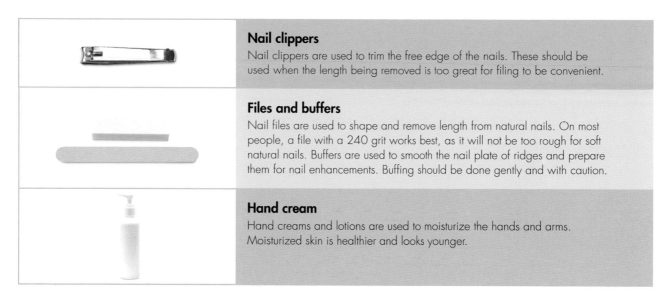

Nail clippers
Nail clippers are used to trim the free edge of the nails. These should be used when the length being removed is too great for filing to be convenient.

Files and buffers
Nail files are used to shape and remove length from natural nails. On most people, a file with a 240 grit works best, as it will not be too rough for soft natural nails. Buffers are used to smooth the nail plate of ridges and prepare them for nail enhancements. Buffing should be done gently and with caution.

Hand cream
Hand creams and lotions are used to moisturize the hands and arms. Moisturized skin is healthier and looks younger.

Product Ingredients

Some chemicals used to optimize product performance have been shown to carry health risks. There are many options on the market now, enabling consumers to exercise some control over levels of exposure to chemicals. Always read the label and stay informed about ingredients.

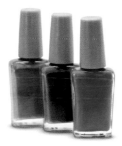

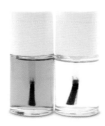

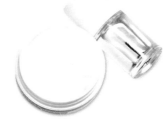

THE BIG THREE
Formaldehyde, toluene, and dibutyl phthalate (DBP), the 'Big 3', are a group of chemicals implicated in birth defects and certain cancers. For this reason, some companies exclude them from their nail polish formulas. Most brands are now 3-free but always check the label to be sure. Pregnant women and children should avoid using polishes and products that are not 3-free.

TOP COAT AND NAIL TREATMENT
Top coats that contain DBP or toluene, referred to as 2-free, perform better on nail art, as smearing is minimal. 3-free top coats are thinner and give a shiny finish, but you may need to wait for your nail art to dry completely and then apply several coats to achieve a smooth surface. Some nail treatments contain formaldehyde. This helps make nails stronger, but over time, can cause brittleness. Formaldehyde-free nail treatment formulas are available.

CREAMS AND OILS
Hand creams, cuticle oils, and cuticle creams containing natural oils and butters are a great choice because they are most similar to natural body oils. Jojoba oil is molecularly small enough to penetrate the nail plate, encouraging a healthy moisture balance and increased flexibility. Shea butter is renowned for having measurable healing qualities that are particularly good for the skin.

Nail Art Tools

Many people struggle to create beautiful nail art because they lack the correct tools. For the tutorials in this book, you will need a few industry-specific implements as well as some common household items. You can find these tools at chemists, beauty supply shops, or online.

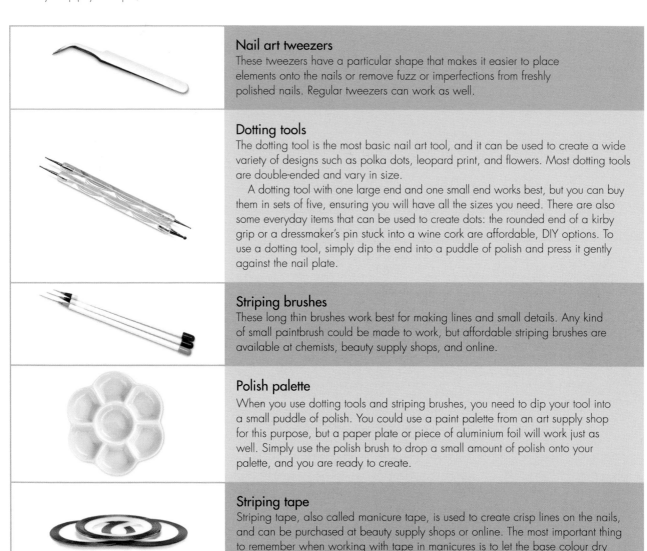

Nail art tweezers
These tweezers have a particular shape that makes it easier to place elements onto the nails or remove fuzz or imperfections from freshly polished nails. Regular tweezers can work as well.

Dotting tools
The dotting tool is the most basic nail art tool, and it can be used to create a wide variety of designs such as polka dots, leopard print, and flowers. Most dotting tools are double-ended and vary in size.

A dotting tool with one large end and one small end works best, but you can buy them in sets of five, ensuring you will have all the sizes you need. There are also some everyday items that can be used to create dots: the rounded end of a kirby grip or a dressmaker's pin stuck into a wine cork are affordable, DIY options. To use a dotting tool, simply dip the end into a puddle of polish and press it gently against the nail plate.

Striping brushes
These long thin brushes work best for making lines and small details. Any kind of small paintbrush could be made to work, but affordable striping brushes are available at chemists, beauty supply shops, and online.

Polish palette
When you use dotting tools and striping brushes, you need to dip your tool into a small puddle of polish. You could use a paint palette from an art supply shop for this purpose, but a paper plate or piece of aluminium foil will work just as well. Simply use the polish brush to drop a small amount of polish onto your palette, and you are ready to create.

Striping tape
Striping tape, also called manicure tape, is used to create crisp lines on the nails, and can be purchased at beauty supply shops or online. The most important thing to remember when working with tape in manicures is to let the base colour dry completely before applying the tape.

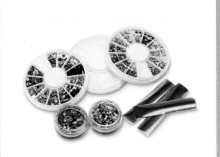

Studs, stones, glitter, sequins, and foils

A wide variety of elements can be applied to your nails. Studs, rhinestones, nail charms, tiny sequins, and loose glitter can be purchased at beauty supply shops and online, as well as at general craft shops. While these products are specifically designed for use on the nail, there are many other things that you could experiment with. For example, if you want to create something bold and wild, look out for small trinkets that could be stuck to the nail as a charm.

Nail foils are metallic foil strips with a clear backing to make them easy to apply to the nail. They are available in solid colours and designs. While there are a variety of ways to use foils, you must use a foil adhesive if you want to apply the foils smoothly to the entire nail.

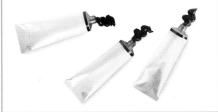

Acrylic paint

For nail artists who work in very fine detail, acrylic paint may work better than traditional nail polish. Although it is not designed specifically for nail art, acrylic paint is water-soluble and safe to use on nails. It dries quickly, stays where you apply it, and appears shiny when finished with a top coat. Affordable acrylic paints can be purchased at any art or craft supply shop.

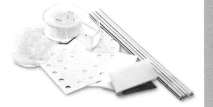

Household items

Many of the tools used in the tutorials in this book you probably already have at home, such as drinking straws, cosmetic sponges, plastic wrap, hole reinforcement stickers, and clear adhesive tape.

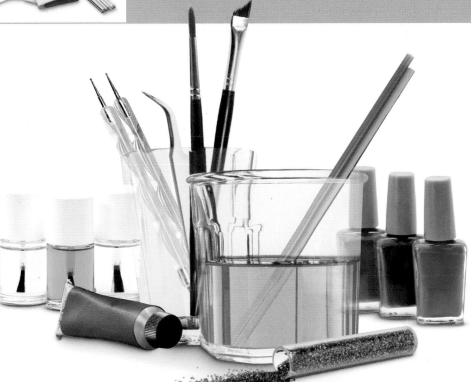

Manicure Step by Step

The perfect nail art manicure looks its best when it starts with healthy, well maintained nails. By implementing a few simple habits into your daily routine and adopting healthy manicure techniques, you will see a difference in your nails in just a few days. To stay on top of your nail care routine and create strong, beautiful nails, give your nails a bi-weekly manicure at home.

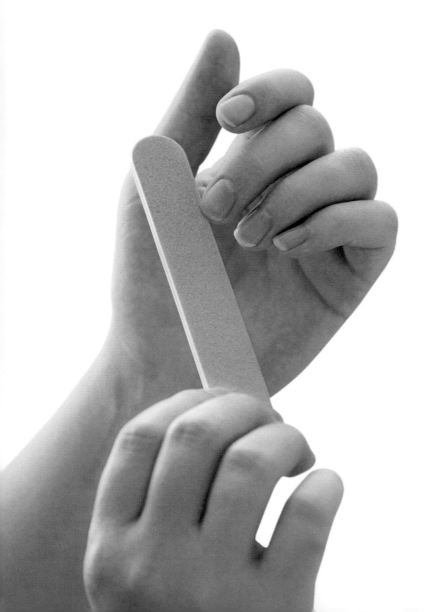

MATERIALS

Nail file

Cuticle remover

Cuticle pusher

Cuticle oil

Hand cream

Cotton wool balls

Nail treatment

Base coat

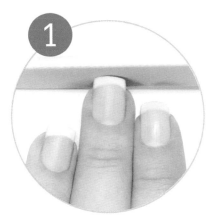

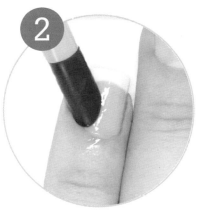

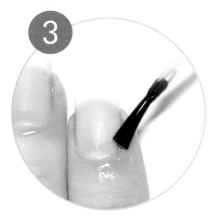

File your nails to the desired length and shape. File in one direction at a time and avoid using a sawing motion. A gentle, high-grit file is always best on natural nails.

Apply a cuticle remover to your nail plate. Using a cuticle pusher, gently ease back your cuticles. Do not push too hard or force the eponychium back. Only if needed, use nippers to remove the sticky cuticle tissue that may cling to the nail plate. Never cut your eponychium – it is living tissue.

Apply cuticle oil to the base of the nail and massage it into your eponychium and nails.

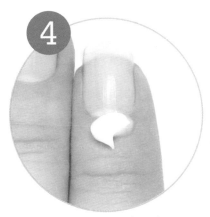

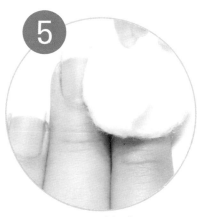

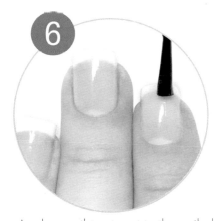

Apply a moisturizing hand cream to your eponychium and massage it into the base of your nail plate, the ends of your fingers, and into your hands.

Use a cotton wool ball to remove any excess hand cream that has not been absorbed, leaving you with clean, natural nails.

Apply a nail treatment to the nail plate. Most also double as a base coat, but some manicurists will use both products in a manicure. Base coat not only helps prevent staining, it helps polish adhere to the nail plate.

Polish Step by Step

Polishing your nails does not need to be a stressful experience. In fact, once you have grown accustomed to using a proper polishing technique, you will probably find it a relaxing and enjoyable ritual. The steps shown here will produce a long-lasting, beautiful base for your nail art. When following the tutorials outlined in this book, always use a base coat, a top coat, and the clean-up technique outlined here.

MATERIALS

Base coat

Nail polish

Top coat

Clean-up brush

Acetone

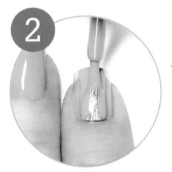

Apply base coat to each nail, covering the entire nail plate. Let them dry for a few minutes.

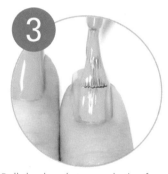

Press the polish brush on to your nail plate, close to the cuticle but not touching it. Repeat if needed to get closer to the eponychium.

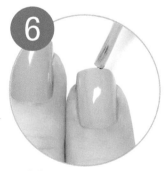

Pull the brush towards the free edge of the nail, creating a stroke of polish.

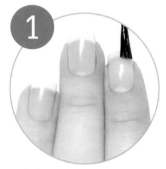

Using a similar method, apply a brush stroke to the right side of your nail.

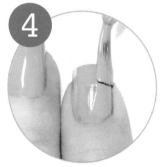

Repeat step 4 on the left side of your nail plate.

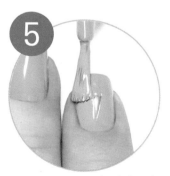

Carefully run the brush along the free edge of your nail, sealing the tip of your nail plate.

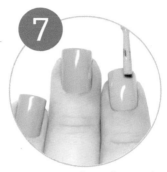

Repeat steps 2 through 6 with a second coat of polish.

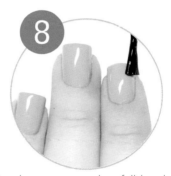

Apply top coat with a full brush and a light hand.

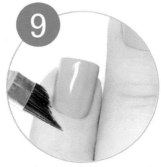

Use a clean-up brush dipped in acetone to lift off excess polish from your skin or cuticle.

Gel Polish Manicures

Gel polish is longer lasting than traditional polish, offering up to two weeks of shiny colour. You can now buy gel sets at a beauty supply shop or online to use at home. For the best results follow the directions closely and only use the products provided in the gel manicure set that you buy.

PREPARING FOR A GEL MANICURE

Gel manicures start with the same preparation as a regular manicure. Start with natural, clean nails. Gently push your eponychium back, clean your nails of excess cuticle tissue, and shape your free edge.

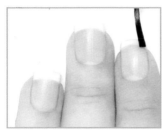

For the gel to adhere to the nail properly, you need to dehydrate your nail plate. The dehydrator shown here (above right) uses a brush-on formula. Some sets will also instruct you to buff your nail plate to remove shine; if so, do this gently and with caution.

Gel polish is generally thicker than regular polish. There is a learning curve when you begin working with it, so read the instructions carefully. For example, to prevent bubbles or lifting, you must apply thin coats of gel.

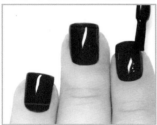

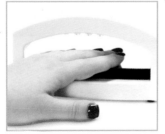

CURING THE GEL

The biggest investment in doing home gel manicures is a UV or LED lamp. Gel needs exposure to such light or it will never dry. UV lamps are generally cheaper, but take two minutes, on average, to cure one coat of gel polish. LED lamps are more expensive, but they take only 30 seconds to cure a layer of polish, and the bulbs rarely need replacing.

DOING NAIL ART WITH GEL

Nail art can be done using gel polish, but be sure to remember to cure each colour you apply before layering something over it. Creating nail art using striping tape is especially convenient with gel polish because the polish is totally dry once it has been cured, reducing drying time.

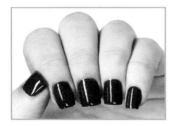

Nail Art Styles

This book features 77 nail art designs, but there are literally thousands of possibilities within these pages. By changing the colours or polish finishes used in the tutorials, you can change the entire look of a design and make it appropriate for any social occasion or outfit. You can also combine designs to create unique manicures by layering different elements together or painting different designs on to each nail.

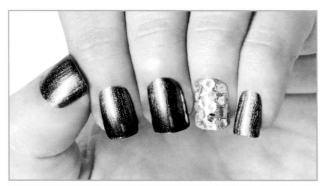

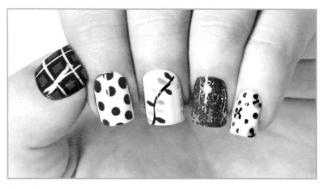

Skittle Manicures

A different design on each nail, in a similar colour family or theme, is known as a 'skittle' manicure. The Christmas skittle manicure (above) includes five separate designs on a similar theme accomplished in a variety of polishes. Other skittle variations include one design done in five different colours.

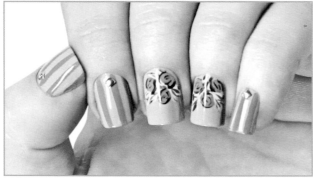

The Accent Nail

The simplest way to put two designs together is with an accent nail or two. To create accent nails, one or two nails are polished differently from the others and this is usually done on the nail of the ring finger or middle finger. Commonly, an accent nail is paired with a coordinating solid colour on the other nails, but two nail art designs could be used as well. A disco ball accent nail (top) really pops against a solid shimmery blue manicure.

Vertical stripes, nail studs, and detailed roses come together in this beautiful double accent nail manicure (above). The two designs are nothing alike, but when done in the same colour family, the result is a cohesive look.

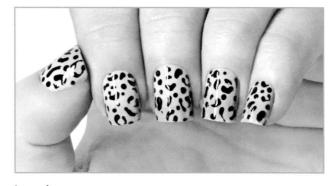

Layering

Some nail art designs, like this gradient and leopard print design (above, lend themselves to layering. Gradients, plastic wrap texture, and dry brushing provide great bases for layering on a black leopard print, zebra stripes, or a striping tape manicure.

3D Elements

3D elements can create a wide variety of manicures. If you want a look that's delicate and feminine or edgy and bold, you can achieve almost anything using 3D elements. As this style of manicure does not require any freehand skill, it is an excellent way to get started with nail art.

Whether you are working with nail studs, loose glitter, sequins, rhinestones, or nail charms, the application is similar. Depending on how long you want your manicure to last, you can apply elements with nail adhesive or glue or simply use top coat.

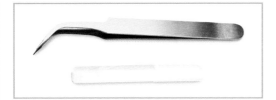

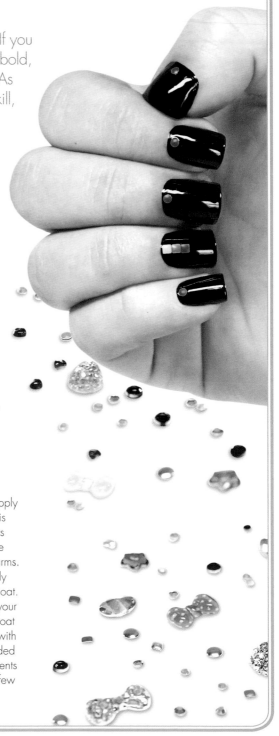

NAIL ART TWEEZERS AND GLUE

To apply 3D elements to your nails for extended wear, apply a drop of nail glue or adhesive to a dry manicure. Use nail art tweezers to place the 3D element in the drop of adhesive. Hold in place until the adhesive begins to dry. If desired, you can apply a layer of thick top coat over small 3D elements, such as studs or rhinestones, for added hold. Nail glue or adhesive generally requires soaking in acetone for removal.

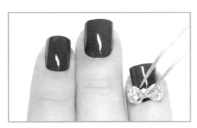

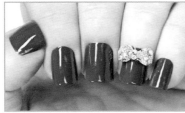

TOP COAT

For a gentler option, you can apply 3D elements using top coat. This works best with smaller elements such as studs, rhinestones, loose glitter, nail sequins, or small charms. Let your manicure dry completely and then apply a layer of top coat. Use nail art tweezers to apply your 3D elements onto the wet top coat and let dry. Seal everything in with a thick layer of top coat for added hold. Generally, small 3D elements applied this way will last for a few days with regular wear.

Polish Removal

Regular nail polish is easily removed with acetone, a solvent commonly used in nail salons because of its effectiveness. Acetone quickly dissolves nail polish and removes it from your nails and skin, limiting the amount of time you are exposed to it. Acetone produces strong fumes, however, and these can lead to headaches and dizziness with over-exposure. Acetone-free polish removers are also available, as well as moisturizing acetone-based formulas that are less harsh. Acetone-free removers still contain chemical solvents, so should not be over-used.

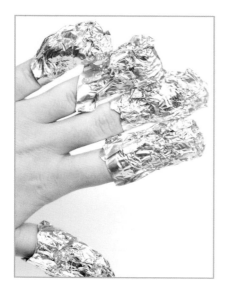

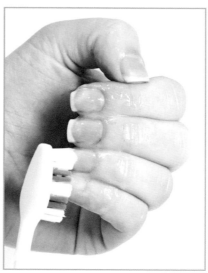

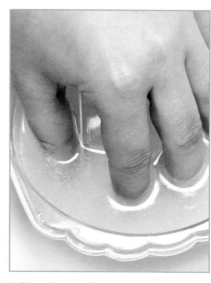

The Foil Method

For gel or tough-to-remove glitter polishes, the foil method is a great option. Soak a cotton wool ball in pure acetone and place it directly on the nail plate. Wrap the entire fingertip securely in a piece of aluminium foil to stop the acetone evaporating. Allow 5 minutes to remove a glitter manicure or 15 minutes for a gel manicure. The polish should slide off the nail when the foil is pulled off. If gel polish is not removed after 15 minutes, apply a fresh, acetone-soaked cotton wool ball and rewrap for 5 minutes. Repeat until the gel slides off the nail plate with the foil.

Stain removal

Certain shades of polish, especially bold blues and greens, are notorious for staining nails. There are a variety of products available that help remove these, but there are some easy home remedies you can try. If you remove your polish to find your nail plates tinted, try scrubbing them with whitening toothpaste – the same ingredients that remove stains from your teeth can remove fresh stains from your nails. You can also try scrubbing them with a paste made of bicarbonate of soda and water. It is a good idea to keep an old toothbrush specifically for this purpose.

Whitening soaks

Older, hard-to-remove stains may require more than a simple scrub. Whitening soaks are available at most beauty supply shops, or you can create your own version with lemon juice and water. Before soaking, gently buff your nails using a high-grit buffer to remove some of the surface staining – a 240-grit nail buffer works well on healthy natural nails. Add several drops of lemon juice to warm water in a bowl or manicure dish and soak your nails for 10–15 minutes. For ready-made whitening soaks, always follow the instructions on the packet.

Pedicures and Toenail Art

Just as manicuring is the art of caring for and beautifying the hands, a pedicure takes care of the feet. Pedicures are luxurious and can be extremely relaxing. Toenails and feet are cared for following a similar procedure as for fingernails and hands.

Soaking

Pedicures begin with the soaking of the feet. This helps to soften the skin and cuticles and is extremely relaxing. Fill a large bowl with warm water (or run some water into the bathtub) and add a foot soak mixture or bath salts. Soak your feet for at least 10 minutes. Remove your feet from the water and pat dry.

Nail Care

A basic pedicure involves shaping the toenails and caring forthe cuticles just as you would do in a manicure. Toenails should be clipped and filed as straight across as possible to avoid ingrowing nails. Once the nails and cuticles are in good shape, you are ready to take care of the rest of your feet.

Scrubs

Pedicure scrubs contain sugar, salt, or other exfoliators to help remove rough dead skin. Apply a liberal amount to your foot and massage it in with damp hands, concentrating on the heel and ball of the foot. Use a foot file or pumice stone to smooth rough areas. Rinse, pat dry, and repeat with your other foot.

Moisturizing

Massage moisturizer into your feet, again focusing on the dry areas as well as the cuticles and tips of the toes. Remove any moisturizer from the nail plate using a cotton wool ball soaked in nail polish remover. Always use a base coat, top coat, and proper clean-up technique when polishing your toenails.

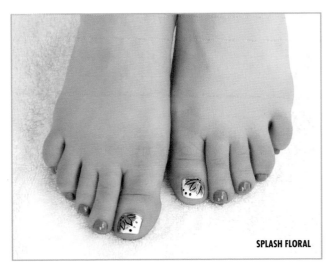

SPLASH FLORAL

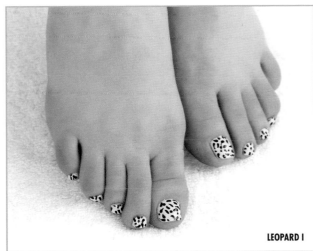

LEOPARD I

Nail Art for Your Toes

Many of the nail art designs in this book can be adapted for the toenails with a bit of creativity. For some designs, it works best to feature the pattern on the big toe and polish the other toenails in a coordinating solid colour, as shown in the Splash Floral pedicure (above). For other designs, all five toenails can feature nail art, though it may be difficult to fit detailed patterns on very small toenails. The Leopard I design (above) makes for a great eye-catching pedicure. Polka dots, florals, and animal print designs are the most popular choices for toenails, but the possibilities are truly unlimited.

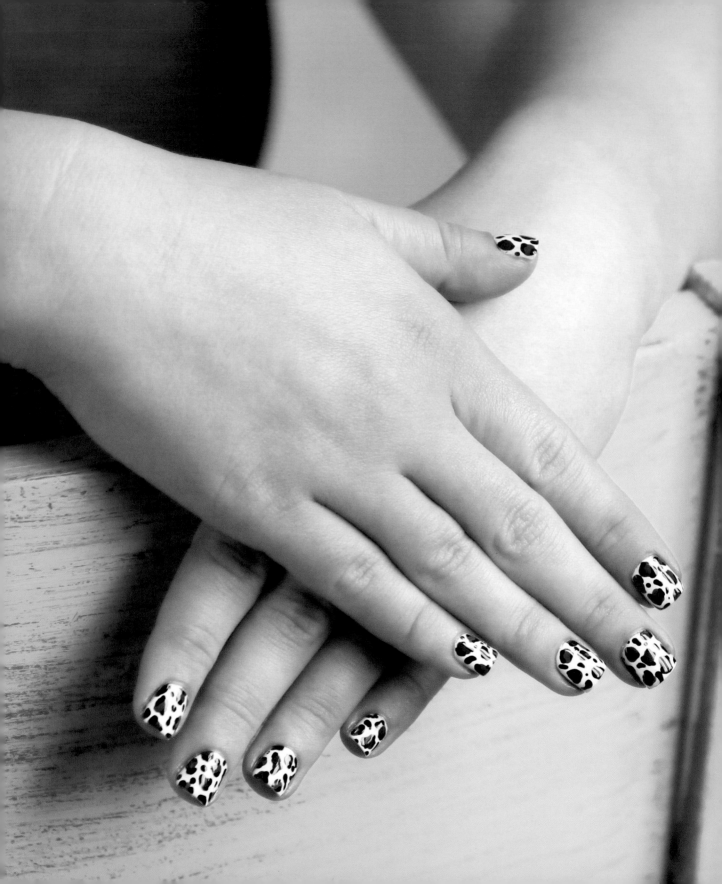

Simple
Designs

There are countless nail art designs that can be created using just a few basic implements, including striping brushes, dotting tools, and tape. Even budding nail artists can confidently work with polka dots and stripes. This section covers 30 manicures that use these basic tools, as well as a few common household items. Practise until you have mastered the techniques in this section, and you will be well prepared to move on to more complex designs.

Classic Dotticure

Nail art designs using polka dots can be feminine, classic, or edgy, depending on the colour palette you choose. Using a dotting tool, dots are easy to create and master. A simple black and white colour scheme creates a look that is perfect any time of year.

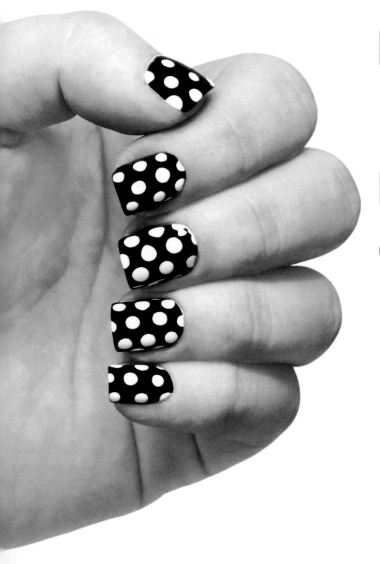

MATERIALS

Dotting tool
Polish palette

POLISH COLOURS

Black   White

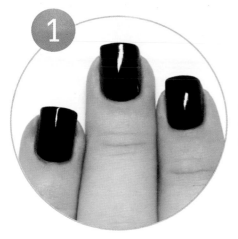

1

Polish your nails with
black polish. Let them
dry for a few minutes.

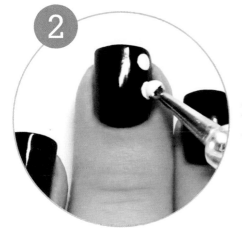

2

Dip your dotting tool into
a small pool of white polish.
With gentle pressure, press
the dotting tool against your
nail to create a dot.

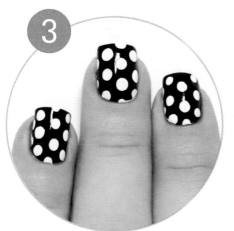

3

Continue creating dots on all
nails in a staggered pattern.

Tip

The dotting tool is
one of the most versatile
nail art tools. In a simple
dotticure, your dots
can be staggered, set
in a line, or randomly
placed round the nail.
Once you are comfortable
with basic dots, there are
many other designs you
can create using just
your dotting tool,
including leopard print
and floral patterns.

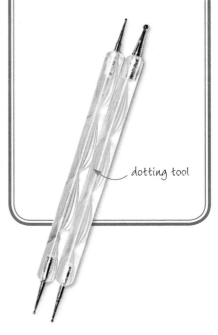

dotting tool

Dotty French

Perhaps the most classic of all nail art techniques is the French tip. It's perfect for formal occasions in its original form, but with a few polka dots, it becomes a fun manicure that can be worn any time. Using tape will help you achieve a perfect edge.

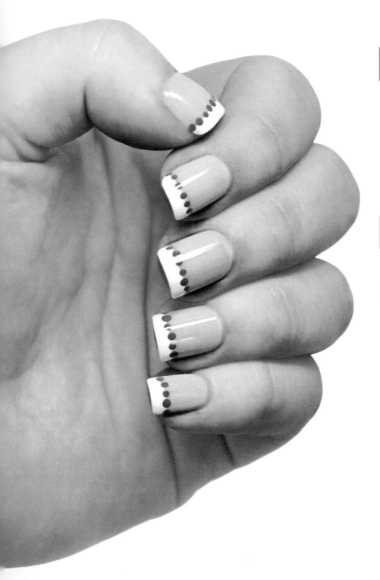

MATERIALS

Tape

Dotting tool

Polish palette

POLISH COLOURS

Sheer pink   White   Pink

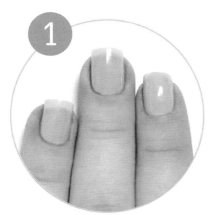

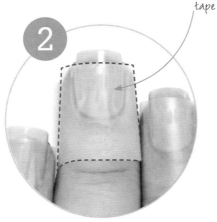

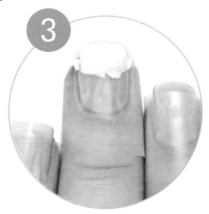

Polish your nails in a sheer pink shade and allow them to dry completely.

Apply a piece of clear adhesive tape to each nail, leaving the very tip of the nail exposed.

On just one nail, apply a white polish where the nail is exposed, creating the French tip.

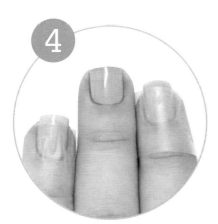

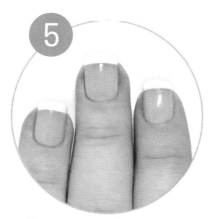

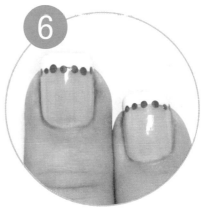

Immediately after applying the white tip, carefully remove the tape from the nail.

Follow steps 3 and 4 to create white tips on the rest of your nails.

Dip your dotting tool into a puddle of pink polish and make dots along the line where the sheer pink and white polishes meet.

Half-Moons

A truly vintage design, the half-moon manicure is extremely versatile. Use contrasting colours or finishes to create something subtle, or something flashy on your fingertips.

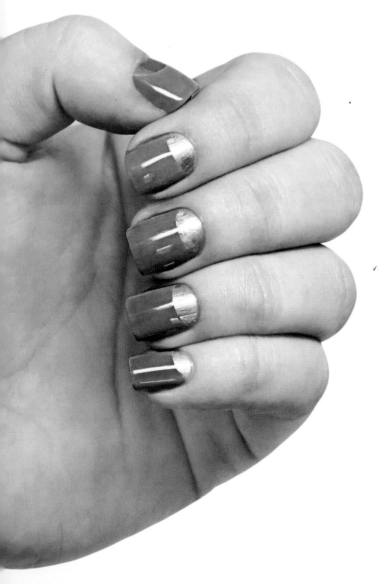

MATERIALS

Hole reinforcement stickers

Scissors

POLISH COLOURS

Gold   Pink

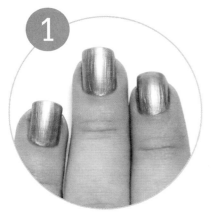

Use scissors to snip open each hole-punch reinforcement sticker. This makes them easier to work with.

Polish your nail in the colour you want your half-moon to be. Here, it will be metallic gold.

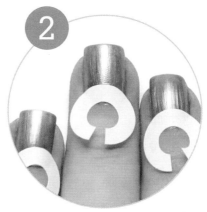

Once the gold polish is quite dry, apply a sticker to the base of each nail, covering a 'half-moon' shape.

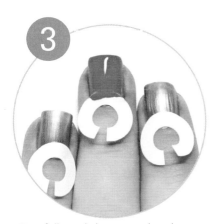

Carefully polish one nail with pink polish.

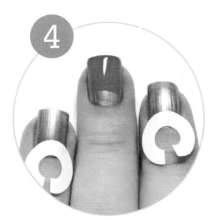

Straight after polishing your nail, gently lift off the sticker.

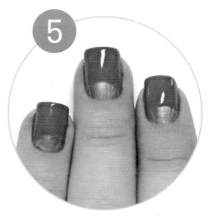

Repeat steps 4 and 5 on the rest of your nails, completing the half-moon manicure.

Leopard I

Once you have mastered painting dots with your dotting tool, leopard print is an easy next step. Whether you use funky bright colours or traditional earthy tones, the final result is always eye-catching.

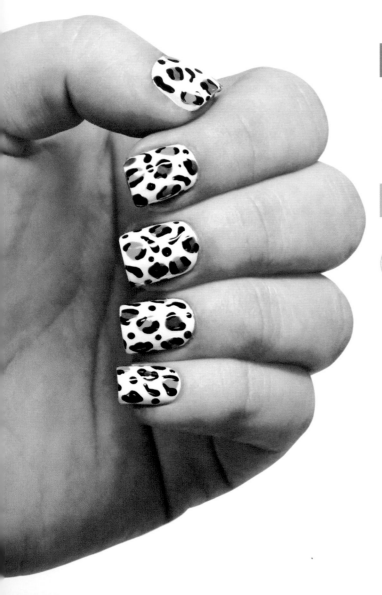

MATERIALS

Dotting tool

Polish palette

POLISH COLOURS

White   Purple   Blue   Black

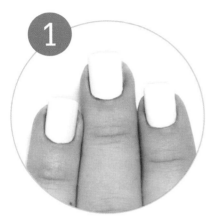

Polish your nails with white polish. Let them dry for a few minutes.

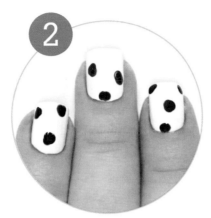

Use your dotting tool to apply a few small 'leopard spots' in purple on each nail. They should be irregularly shaped, and not perfectly round.

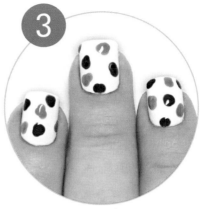

Using the same technique, apply some blue spots. Space them randomly on the nail.

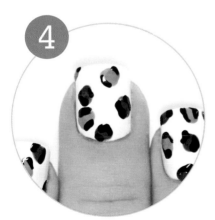

Use your dotting tool to create the black detailing on each spot. C-shapes work well.

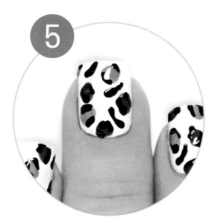

Using gentle pressure and your dotting tool, create a few curved black lines between the coloured spots.

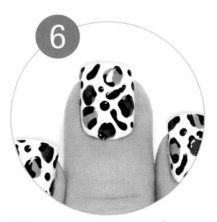

Fill in any empty space with tiny black dots.

Leopard II

Leopard print can be produced in several ways. With this technique, you create the print using only black polish, so you can apply it over a variety of bases: solid colours, gradients, or other textures. The only limit to the effect you can create is your imagination!

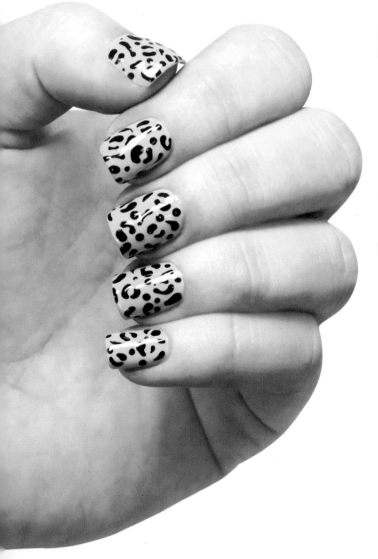

MATERIALS

Dotting tool

Polish palette

POLISH COLOURS

Green   Black

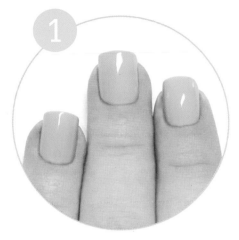

Polish your nails in your base colour, in this example, a bright lime green. Let them dry for a few minutes.

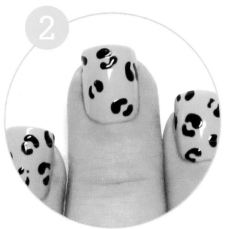

Using a small dotting tool, create leopard spots on your nails in black polish. C-shapes work well.

Leopard print isn't perfect in nature, and it doesn't need to be perfect here either. Your leopard spots can be U-shaped, pairs of C-shapes, or even full circles. Experiment with what you like best. Keep the tip of your dotting tool covered in polish and use only a light pressure when touching the tool to your nail using smooth, sweeping motions.

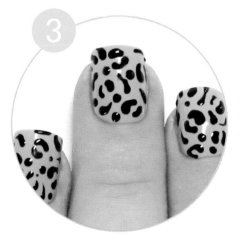

Using only light pressure, create curved black lines and tiny dots with your dotting tool to fill the nail.

Retro Floral

The Retro Floral is one of the easiest floral nail art designs to master. Using only your dotting tool, you can create a whimsically feminine manicure suitable for all young souls, regardless of age.

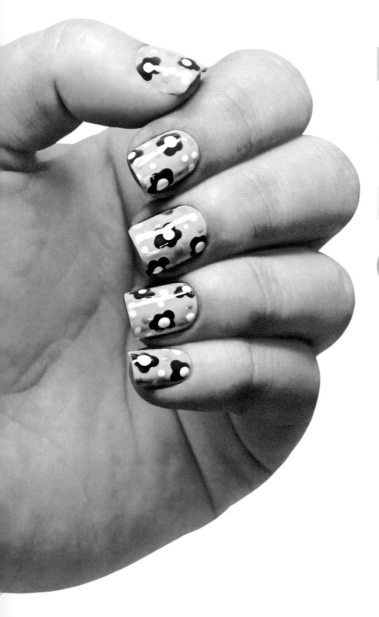

MATERIALS

Dotting tool

Polish palette

POLISH COLOURS

Blue   Purple   White   Green

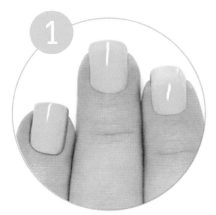

Polish your nails light blue.
Let them dry for a few minutes.

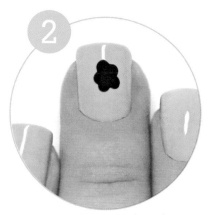

Using your dotting tool, make
five overlapping purple dots in
a circular shape. This should
resemble a flower.

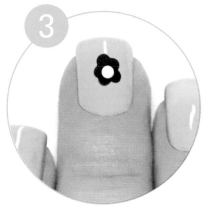

Place a white dot in the centre
of the flower shape.

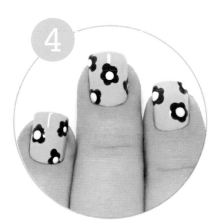

Repeat steps 2 and 3, filling
each nail with flowers. Create
an all-over print by placing
parts of flowers over the edge
of your nails.

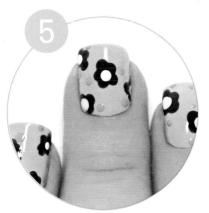

Using the small end of your dotting
tool, place one or two tiny green
dots near each flower.

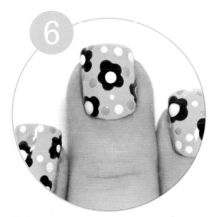

Fill any remaining space with
small white dots.

Vintage Roses

Floral prints represent nail art manicures at their most elegant. This vintage rose design actually appears to be more difficult than it really is. Shades of pink and green add depth to this sophisticated yet simple design.

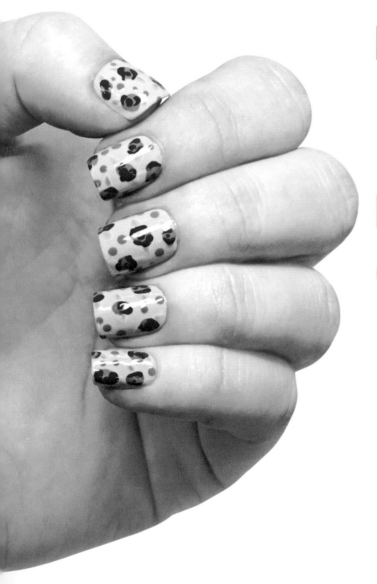

MATERIALS

Dotting tool

Polish palette

Striping brush

POLISH COLOURS

| Pale pink | Light pink | Light green | Green | Magenta |

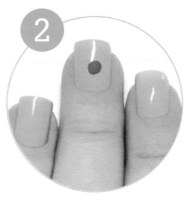

Polish your nails in a shade that complements your skin tone. Let the nails dry for a few minutes.

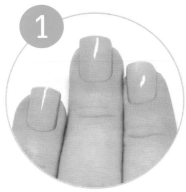

Using your dotting tool, create a round, light pink shape on your nail. This will become a rose.

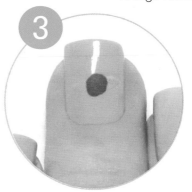

Use your striping brush to draw a light green triangle on either side of the circle.

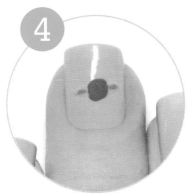

Add a dark green detail line down the centre of each triangle, using your striping brush. These are the leaves.

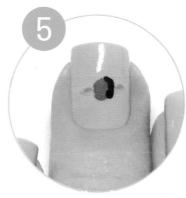

Use the small end of your dotting tool to add a magenta C-shape on one side of the circle.

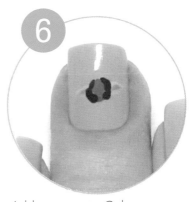

Add a magenta C-shape on the other side of the rose. This should cover where the leaves meet the rose.

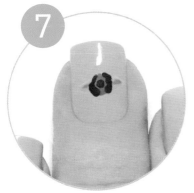

Place a tiny magenta dot in the middle of the circle, finishing the rose.

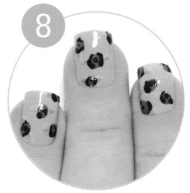

Repeat steps 2 through 7, distributing the roses randomly over all of your nails.

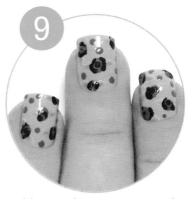

Add several tiny green or pink dots around the flowers to fill in any empty spaces.

Vertical Stripes

Aside from dots, stripes are amongst the most basic nail art elements. On their own or as part of a more complex manicure, stripes can be graphic and eye-catching. A striping brush or a long thin paint brush works best for this technique.

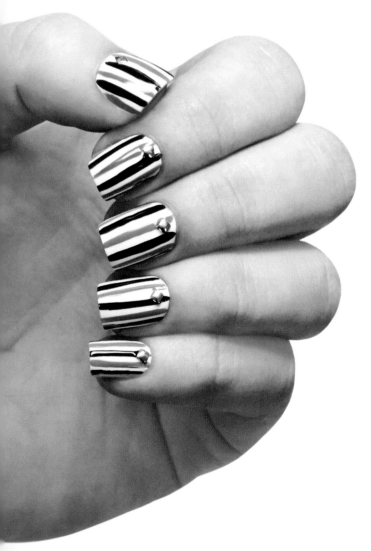

MATERIALS

Striping brush	Top coat
Polish palette	Tweezers
Acetone	Nail studs

POLISH COLOURS

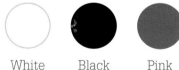

White   Black   Pink

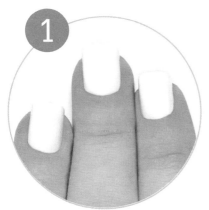

Polish your nails with white polish and let them dry. Place a puddle of black polish on your palette and load your striping brush.

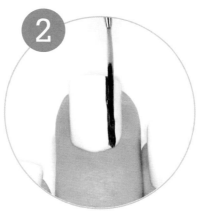

Allow the brush to make contact with your nail near the cuticle and gently pull towards the free edge.

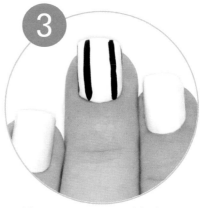

Add one or two more black stripes, spacing them out evenly over your nail.

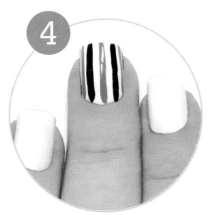

Clean the striping brush with acetone and load it with pink polish. Add pink stripes between the black stripes, allowing some of the base colour to show through.

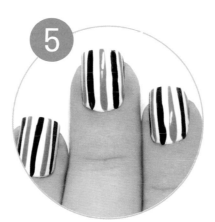

Follow steps 2 through 4 to create black and pink stripes on all of your nails. Let them dry for a few minutes.

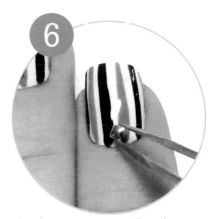

Apply a top coat to all nails. Using your nail art tweezers, place a nail stud in the wet top coat at the base of each nail.

Ruffle Manicure

This abstract and graphic manicure design requires no special tools and works well with a variety of colours and finishes. The ruffle design also makes a great accent nail, as shown in this tutorial. Add a glitter nail to finish the look.

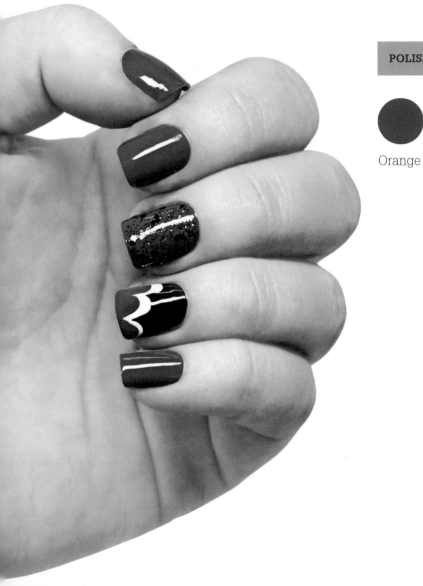

POLISH COLOURS

Orange   Purple   White   Purple glitter

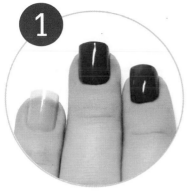

Polish all of your nails except for your ring finger nail with orange polish. Let them dry.

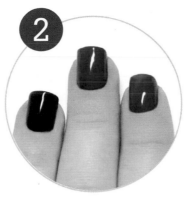

Polish your ring finger nail purple. This will be your ruffle accent nail.

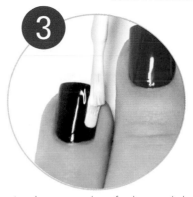

Apply one stroke of white polish near the sidewall of your ring finger nail, starting three-quarters of the way down your nail.

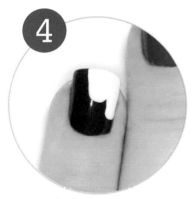

Repeat this technique in the centre of your nail, starting about half-way down the nail and polishing to the free edge.

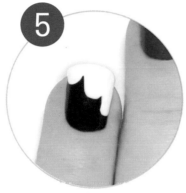

Repeat this technique again, near the other sidewall. Start from about one-quarter of the way down the nail and polish to the free edge.

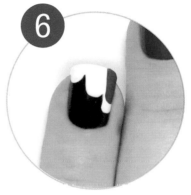

Using the same technique, apply an orange streak over the first white streak, allowing some white to show around the edges.

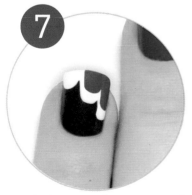

Apply the second orange streak near the middle of the nail. Once again, allow some white to show.

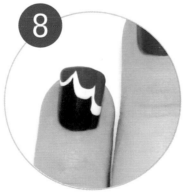

Apply a third orange streak, allowing white to show through at the bottom edge.

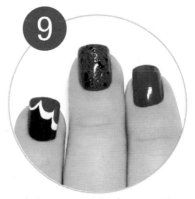

Polish your middle finger with a purple glitter polish, finishing your manicure.

Splatter Manicure

Everyone knows the best crafts are the messy ones. To keep the clean-up to a minimum in this manicure, put pieces of tape around your nails to protect your skin from the polish. You can remove any excess polish with acetone and a clean-up brush, such as an angled eyeliner brush.

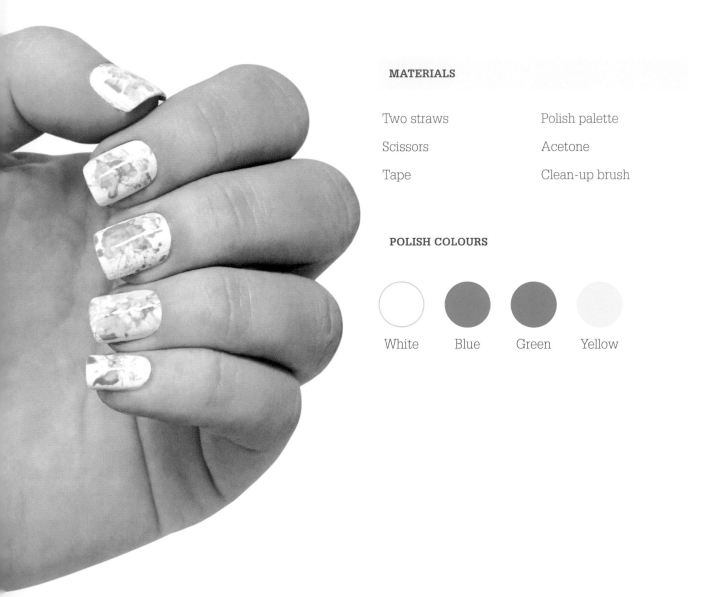

MATERIALS

Two straws

Scissors

Tape

Polish palette

Acetone

Clean-up brush

POLISH COLOURS

White   Blue   Green   Yellow

tape

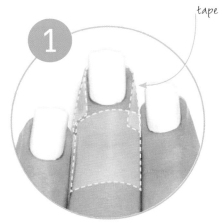

Cut two drinking straws in half and set them aside. Polish your nails white and carefully apply tape around your nails.

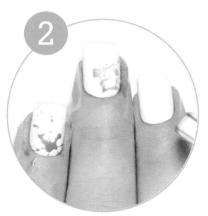

Dip a straw into a puddle of blue polish. Align the straw with your nail and blow through the clean end to add blue splatters to each nail.

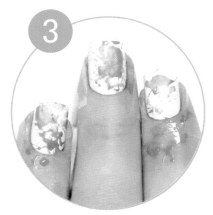

Dip a clean straw into green polish and repeat, adding green splatters to the nails.

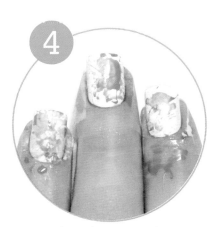

Repeat the splattering technique once again, using another straw and yellow polish.

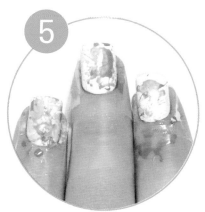

If needed, fill in empty space with splatters in any colour you like.

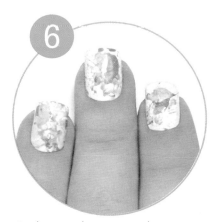

Peel away the tape and remove any excess polish using a clean-up brush soaked in acetone.

Cloud Manicure

This whimsical nail design brings a hint of springtime, and is perfect to wear for a picnic on a sunny day, or even on a dull day that needs a little cheering up. Using only a dotting tool, your nails will look like a blue sky filled with fluffy clouds in minutes.

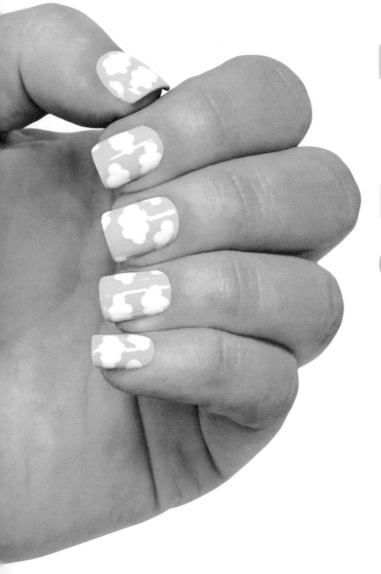

MATERIALS

Dotting tool

Polish palette

POLISH COLOURS

Sky blue   White

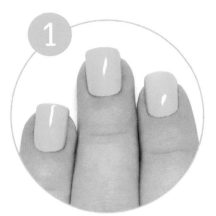

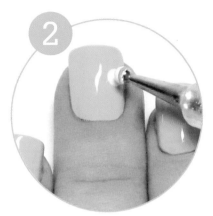

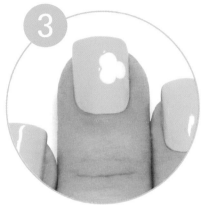

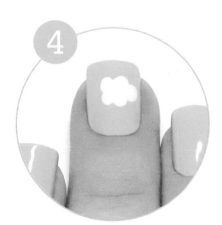

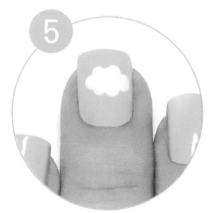

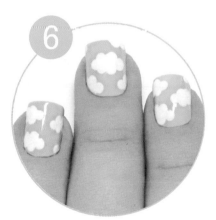

Polish your nails in sky blue polish. Let them dry for a few minutes.

Dip your dotting tool into a puddle of white polish and create a single white dot on your nail.

Create two more white dots that overlap the first one, to begin to build up the cloud shape.

Create two more dots overlapping the dots you made in step 3.

Finish your cloud by adding a single white dot, centred next to and overlapping the dots you made in step 4.

Fill your nails with cloud shapes, spacing them evenly across the entire nail. Create partial clouds that appear to go off the edge of your nail for a complete look.

Deep-V Manicure

This stylish variation on a French manicure is perfect for those who want a formal look but without playing it too safe. Striping tape helps keep the lines crisp and clean, though you could do this freehand if you're confident in your brush skills.

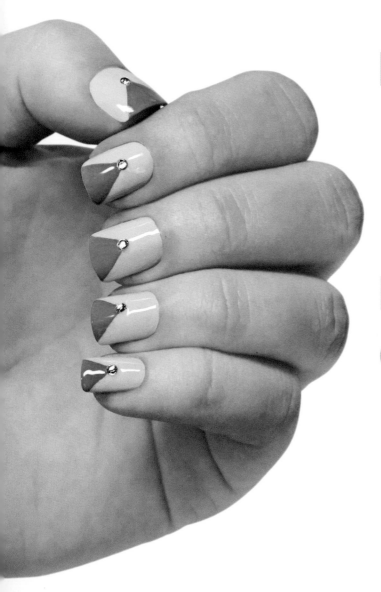

MATERIALS

Striping tape

Striping brush

Top coat

Tweezers

Rhinestones

POLISH COLOURS

Grey   Pink

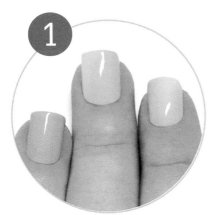

Polish your nails in grey polish. Leave them for a few minutes to dry completely.

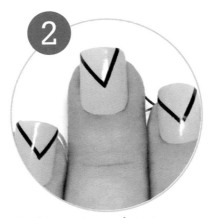

Apply two pieces of striping tape to each nail in a V-shape and press them on to the nail.

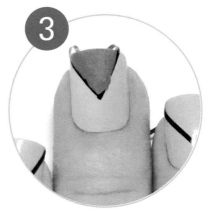

Polish the tip of one nail in pink polish, staying within the lines of the striping tape.

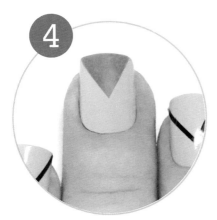

Remove the striping tape. Fix lines with your striping brush if there are any imperfections.

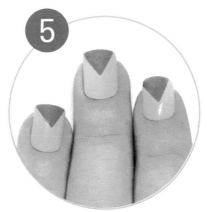

Repeat steps 3 and 4 on all of your nails, one nail at a time. Let them dry completely.

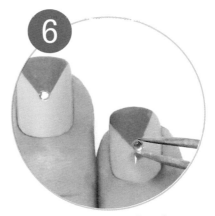

Apply a top coat to all nails. Use tweezers to set a rhinestone into the wet top coat at the apex of each deep V.

Simple Gradient

One of the most popular nail art looks, the simple gradient can add a extra dimension to just about any manicure. Wear a gradient on its own or with nail art layered over the top for a striking textural manicure that is perfect for any occasion.

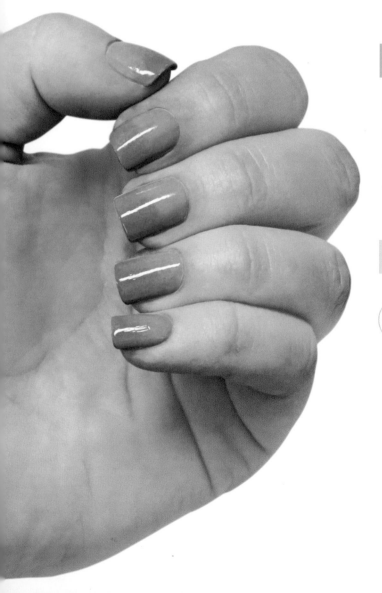

MATERIALS
Cosmetic sponge
Clean-up brush
Acetone
Top coat

POLISH COLOURS

White   Pink   Orange

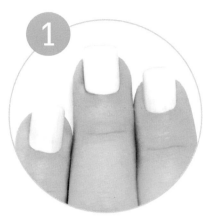

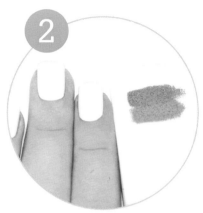

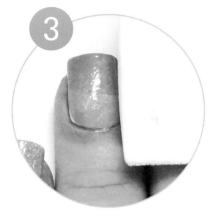

Polish your nails white and let them dry for a few minutes.

Paint side-by-side stripes of the gradient colours (in this case, pink and orange) on to a cosmetic sponge.

Press the polish on to your nails using gentle pressure.

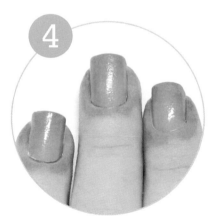

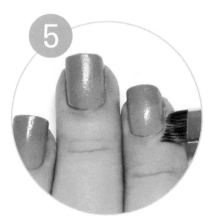

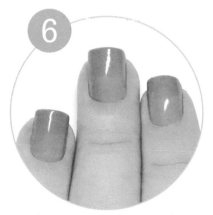

Repeatedly press the polish on to your nails, moving the sponge up and down slightly to blend the colours. Continue pressing until you achieve the gradient effect you desire.

Use acetone and an angled eyeliner brush to remove the excess polish from your skin.

Apply a top coat to your nails to help blend the gradient and finish the look.

Cling Film

Adding textural interest to your manicure can really emphasize the 'wow' factor. Whether you wear this textured look on its own or as a base under beautiful nail art, you will be pleased with how simple it is to achieve.

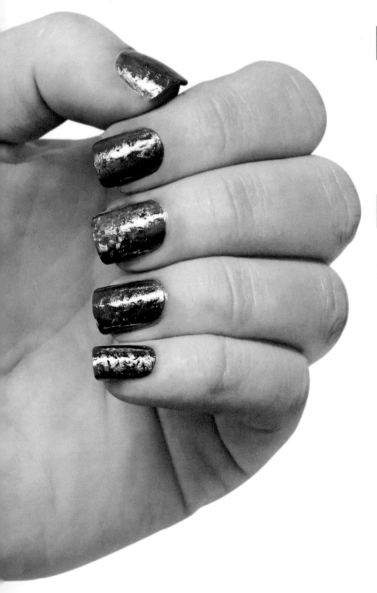

MATERIALS

Cling film

Acetone

Clean-up brush

POLISH COLOURS

Blue   Gold

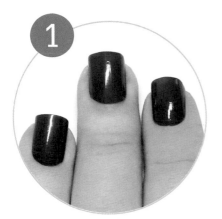

Polish your nails blue. Let them dry for a few minutes.

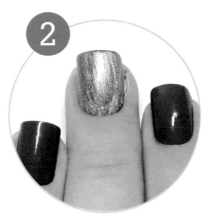

Paint a thick coat of gold polish over the dried blue polish on one nail.

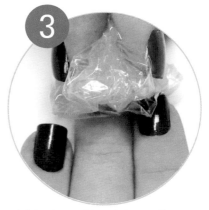

While the gold polish is still wet, press a piece of wrinkled-up cling film on to the nail, lifting some of the gold polish off of it.

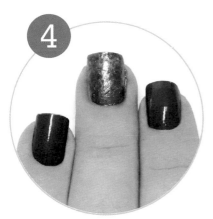

Apply more gold polish in sparse dots and press again with cling film until you achieve the textural effect you want.

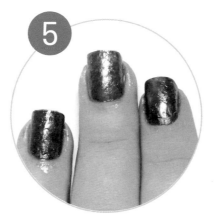

Repeat steps 2 through 4 on your other nails, one at a time.

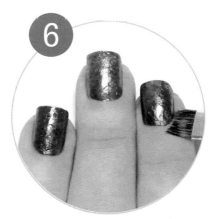

This technique will require cleaning up. Use an angled eyeliner brush soaked in acetone to remove any nail polish from your skin.

Zebra

Animal-print manicures can be feminine yet sassy, and zebra print is no exception. As you become comfortable with the basic method for creating zebra stripes, you will develop your own techniques for letting the stripes flow over the nail.

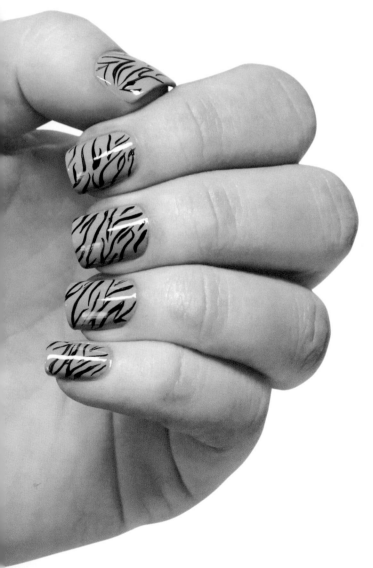

MATERIALS

Striping brush

Polish palette

POLISH COLOURS

Taupe   Black

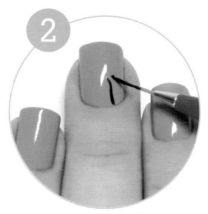

Polish your nails taupe. Let them dry for a few minutes.

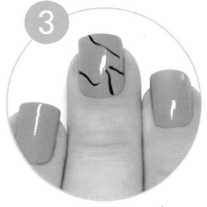

Load your striping brush with black polish or acrylic paint and create a V-shape at the corner of the nail.

Paint two stripes coming in from the opposite side of the nail.

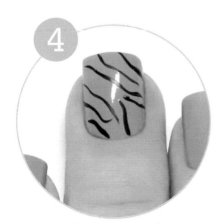

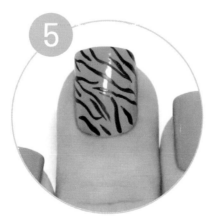

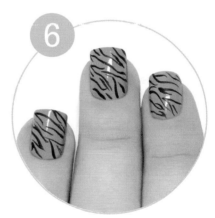

Between the stripes you have just made, paint stripes coming from the same side of the nail as the original V-shape.

Add small lines to a few of the stripes, creating several more V shapes and filling empty space on the nail.

Finish your manicure by repeating steps 2 through 5 on all of your nails, or wear the zebra print as an accent nail.

Laser Manicure

Tape manicures require a lot of patience, but the finished look is always worth the extra effort. This manicure is graphic and eye-catching, and you can use a variety of contrasting colour schemes to make your look really pop!

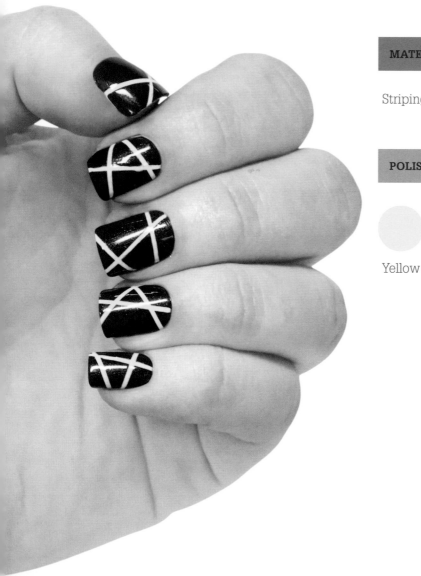

MATERIALS

Striping tape

POLISH COLOURS

Yellow   Red

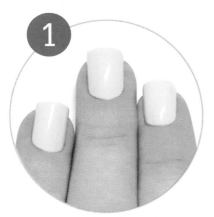

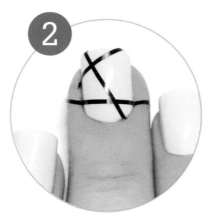

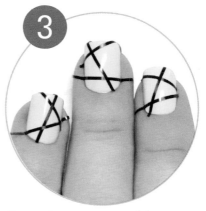

1 Polish your nails yellow. This will be the colour of your laser beams. Let your nails dry for a few minutes.

2 Apply three pieces of striping tape to each nail in an angular pattern.

3 Rotate the orientation of the tape on each nail to create a more interesting finished manicure.

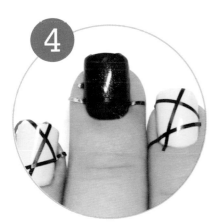

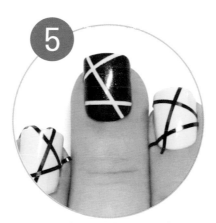

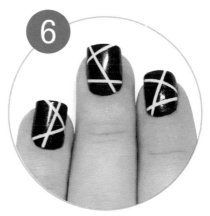

4 Apply red polish all over the nail plate and striping tape on one nail.

5 Straight after polishing, gently remove the striping tape, revealing your design.

6 Repeat steps 4 and 5 on your remaining nails, finishing the manicure.

Dry Brush

If you just cannot decide which polish to wear, use this method to wear them all at once. The resulting textural finish is perfect on its own or as a base under nail art. Using only the polish brush and any combination of colours and finishes, you can create a fascinating range of looks.

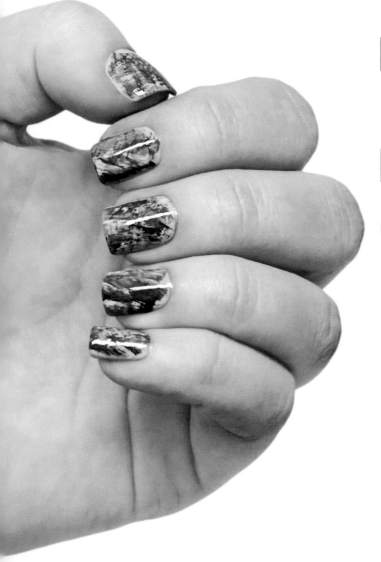

MATERIALS

Kitchen paper

POLISH COLOURS

Beige   Pink   Purple   Blue

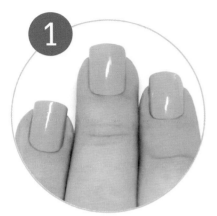

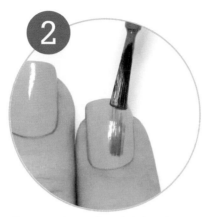

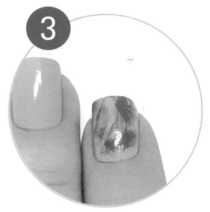

Polish your nails with beige polish. Let them dry for a few minutes.

Remove the pink polish brush from the bottle and wipe nearly all the polish off on a piece of kitchen paper. Gently drag the brush across the nail.

Repeat this all over the nail plate, at varying angles and lengths.

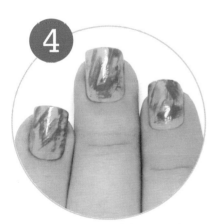

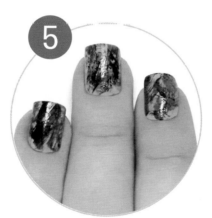

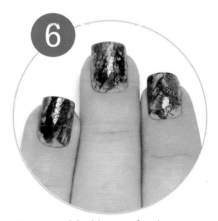

Repeat steps 2 and 3 to apply the pink to all of your nails, using the dry brushing method.

To create a more complex manicure, repeat steps 2 through 4 using a purple polish.

For an added layer of colour, repeat steps 2 through 4 using a blue polish.

Glitter Gradient

Wearing this modern, formal manicure will make you feel like royalty. You can use a cosmetic sponge to apply glitter to your tips, but this tutorial will teach you how to create a true gradient of sparkle using just the polish brush.

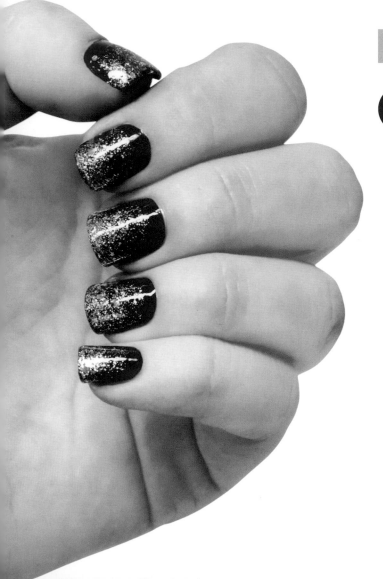

POLISH COLOURS	
Pink	Silver glitter

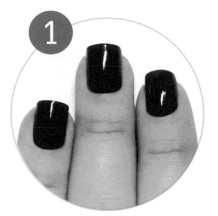

Polish your nails pink. Let them dry for a few minutes.

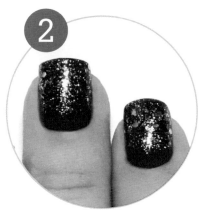

Using the brush from the bottle, apply a thin coat of silver glitter polish. Begin three-quarters down your nail and paint to the tip.

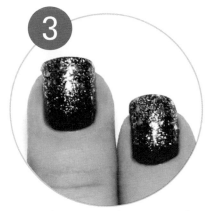

Using the same technique, apply another thin coat of silver glitter polish from half-way down the nail to the tip.

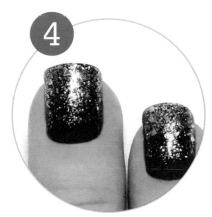

Apply a third thin coat of glitter, from one-quarter of the way down the nail to the tip. Don't let the polish get too thick on the nail.

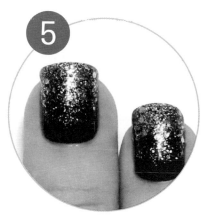

Add a final stroke of glitter polish right at the tip of the nail.

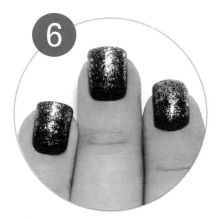

Fill in any space that is in need of glitter to make the gradient flow well.

Sound Wave Manicure

The Sound Wave Manicure is a great way to bring together two of your favourite polish colours. Use this design as a simple, fun accent nail or wear it on all ten nails. Pink and grey are feminine and subtle, but you could also play with bolder contrasting colours.

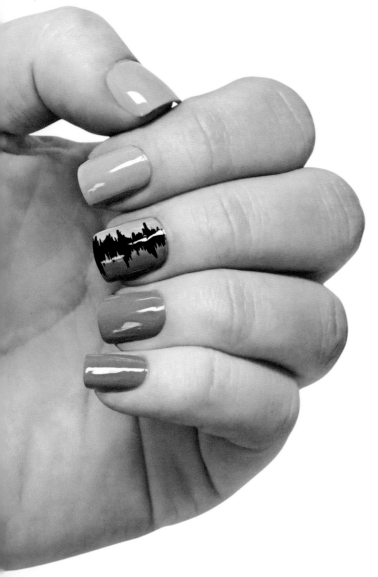

MATERIALS

Tape   Polish palette

Striping brush   Top coat

POLISH COLOURS

Grey   Pink   Black

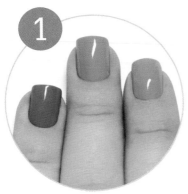

1. Polish your little and ring finger nails pink and your middle finger, index finger, and thumb nails grey. Let dry for a few minutes.

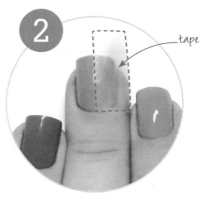

2. Apply a length of tape to your middle finger nail, leaving the half nearest to your ring finger nail exposed.

tape

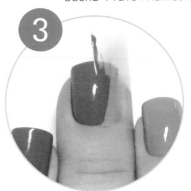

3. Polish the exposed part of your middle finger nail pink.

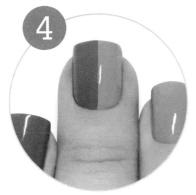

4. Straight after polishing, remove the tape. If your line is not flawless, don't worry. This will be covered up.

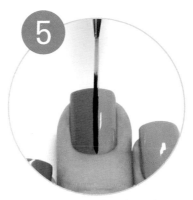

5. Using a striping brush and black polish or acrylic paint, paint a stripe down the centre of the middle finger nail.

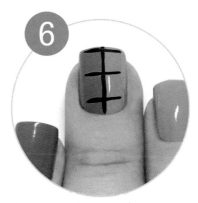

6. Paint three horizontal lines along the length of the first vertical line.

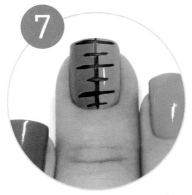

7. Paint three shorter horizontal lines between each of the lines you created in step 6.

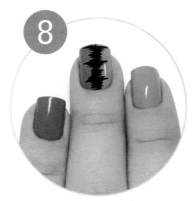

8. Begin painting more lines, creating a symmetric curve on each side of the sound wave.

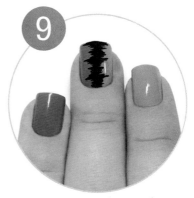

9. Fill in the curve with more lines so the sound wave is solid and nearly symmetrical. Finish with a top coat.

Basic Tape Manicure

There are endless ways you can use tape to create straight lines in your manicures. This design uses tape to create an angled tip with a subtle accent of polka dots. Be creative and you'll be surprised how many designs you can come up with.

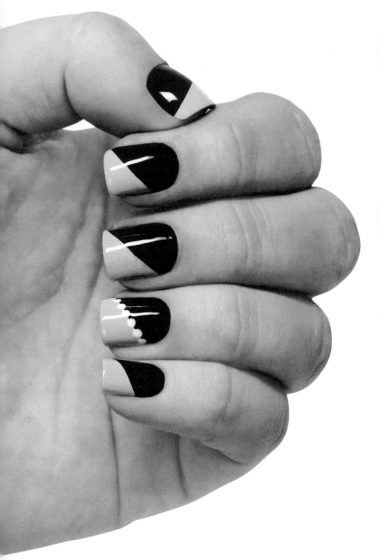

MATERIALS

Tape

Polish palette

Dotting tool

POLISH COLOURS

Turquoise   Red   White

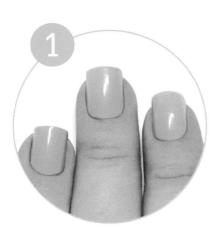

Polish your nails turquoise. Let them dry for a few minutes.

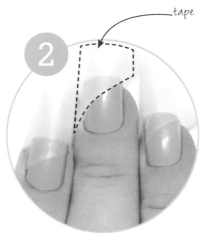

Apply a length of clear adhesive tape to each nail at an angle, covering the tip of the nail.

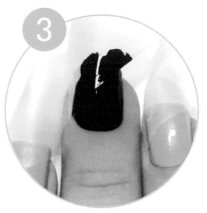

Polish the exposed portion of one nail with red polish.

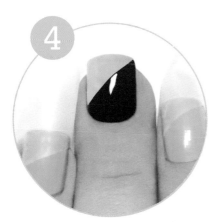

Immediately after applying the red polish, remove the tape. If you let it dry before you peel away the tape, the line won't be as crisp.

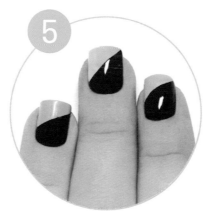

Repeat steps 3 and 4 on all of your nails.

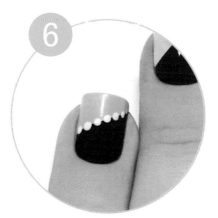

If desired, use your dotting tool to add a few white polka dots on your ring finger nail for an accent nail.

Glitter Frames

Individual pieces of loose glitter can be used to create a striking feature. Carefully placing them around the edge of the nail will accentuate its shape and add the perfect amount of sparkle.

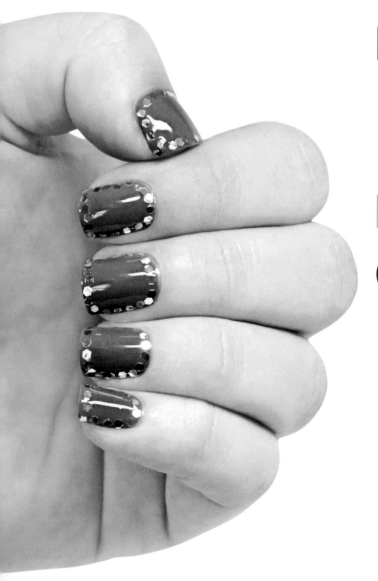

MATERIALS

Top coat (not quick-dry)

Dotting tool

Loose glitter pieces

POLISH COLOURS

Purple

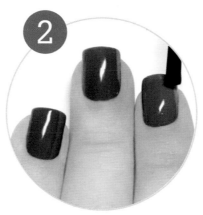

Polish your nails purple. Let them dry for a few minutes.

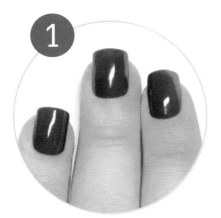

Apply top coat to one nail.

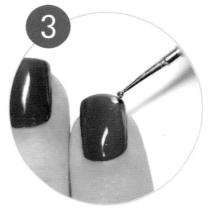

While the nail is wet, use a dotting tool dipped in top coat to pick up a piece of glitter and apply it to your nail, near the free edge.

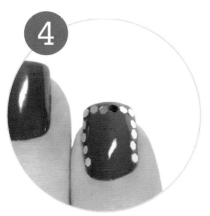

Continue placing glitter pieces along the free edge and down each sidewall.

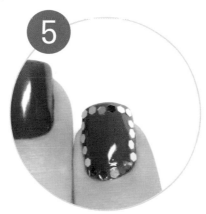

Finish by applying glitter pieces along the curve at the base of your nail.

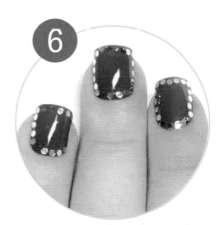

Repeat steps 2 through 5 to place glitter on all nails. Seal the glitter in place with two layers of top coat.

Black Cat

Hallowe'en is the perfect time for a Black Cat manicure. This simple design is interesting because each nail is a bit different, but it comes together into a cohesive seasonal look that is both clever and adorable!

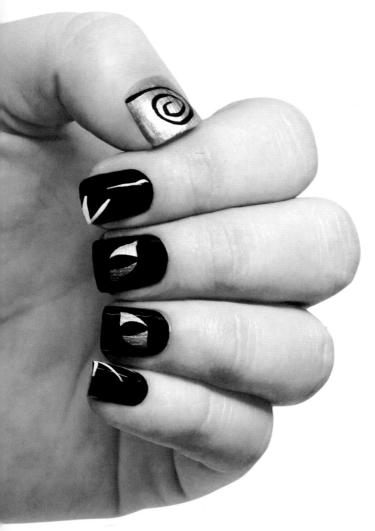

MATERIALS

Striping brush

Polish palette

POLISH COLOURS

Black

Gold

White

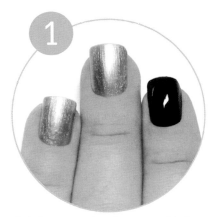

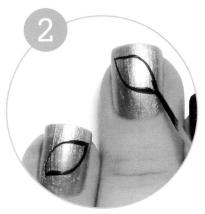

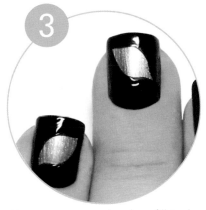

Polish your index finger and little finger nails black. Polish your remaining nails gold. Let them dry for a few minutes.

Using your striping brush and black polish or acrylic paint, create angled leaf-shape eyes on the middle and ring finger nails.

Use your striping brush to fill in the space around the eyes with black polish so that only the leaf shapes are gold.

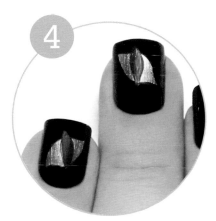

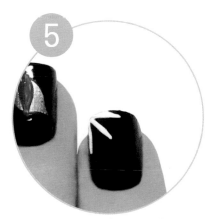

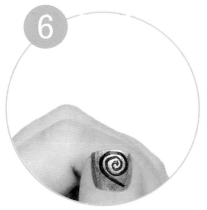

Using your striping brush and black polish or acrylic paint, create pupils in the eyes.

Using white polish or acrylic paint and your striping brush, create three lines coming from the corner of your index and little finger nails. These are the cat's whiskers.

Using black polish or acrylic paint and your striping brush, carefully paint a curly 'tail' on your thumb nail.

Shiny-Matt Manicure

The Shiny-Matt Manicure is a great opportunity to play with contrasting polish finishes. This tutorial features a matt base and a shiny triangular design, but you can use shiny-matt contrast with many designs, such as dots, zebra, and leopard.

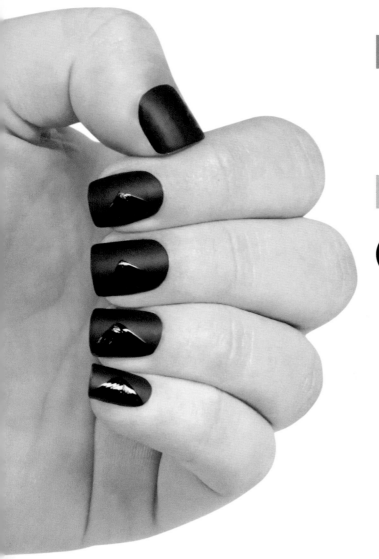

MATERIALS	
Matt top coat	Striping brush
Top coat	Polish palette

POLISH COLOURS

Black

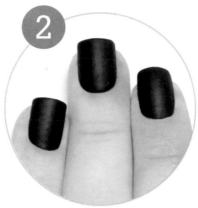

1

Polish your nails black.

2

Apply matt top coat to all of your nails. Let them dry for a few minutes.

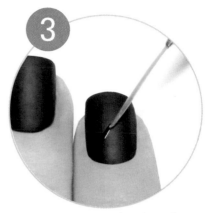

3

Using your striping brush and clear top coat, paint a line from the bottom to the centre of your nail plate.

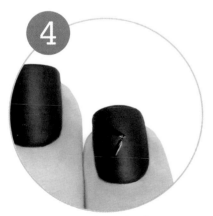

4

Repeat step 3 from the free edge to the centre.

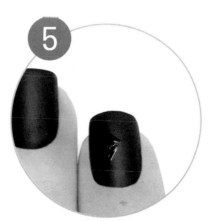

5

Fill in the triangle with clear top coat using your striping brush.

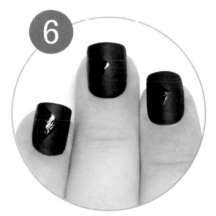

6

Complete steps 3 through 5 on all of your nails for a striking monochromatic look.

Disco Ball

When you have a special occasion and your nails need to look the part, it doesn't get any more glittery than the Disco Ball nail. This design is simple to do, and the sparkle pay-off is enormous! Wear this as a full manicure or as an accent nail.

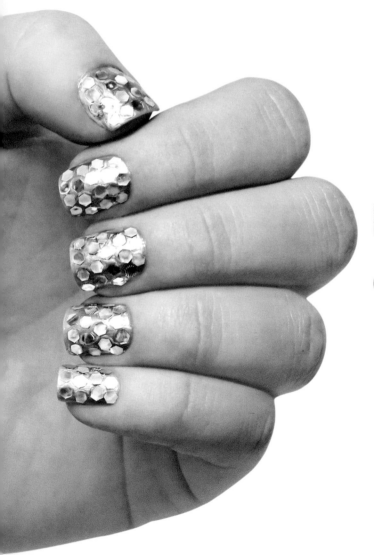

MATERIALS

Top coat (not quick-dry)

Dotting tool

Nail art glitter sequins

POLISH COLOURS

Silver

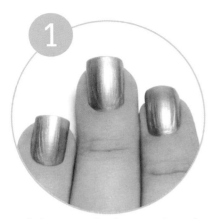

Polish your nails silver. Let them dry for a few minutes.

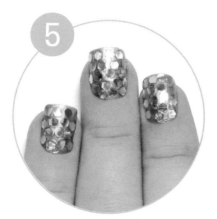

Apply a coat of top coat to one nail.

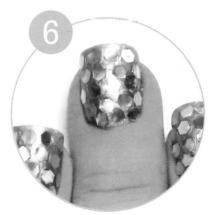

Use a dotting tool dipped in top coat to pick up a glitter sequin and place it on your nail.

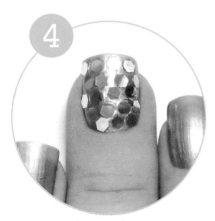

Continue placing glitter sequins on your nail until the nail plate is completely covered.

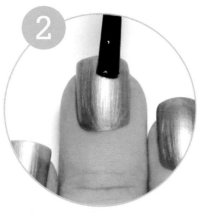

Repeat steps 2 through 4 on all of your nails, completing one nail at a time.

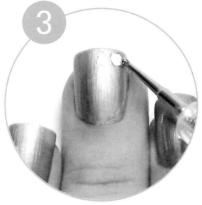

Seal in the glitter sequins with two layers of top coat.

Herringbone

Sometimes less is more. Simply by using straight lines, you can create a striking herringbone design that looks great over any polish colour or finish you choose. You can keep it classic over a neutral base or play it up with a brighter colour, as shown here.

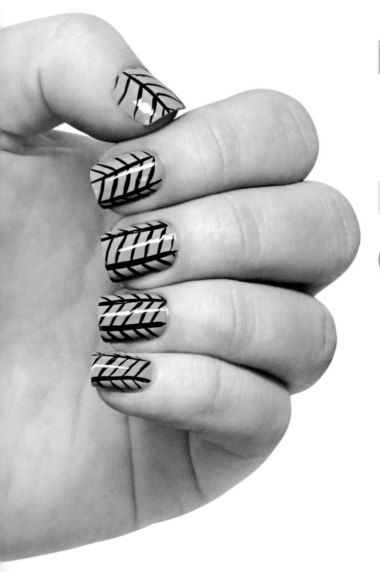

MATERIALS

Striping brush

Polish palette

POLISH COLOURS

Blue   Black

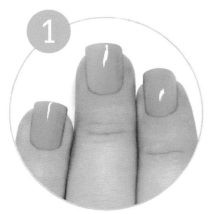

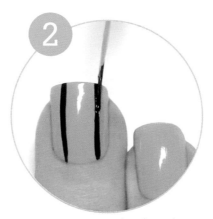

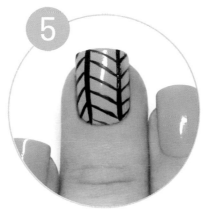

Polish your nails blue. Let them dry for a few minutes.

Using your striping brush and black polish or acrylic paint, paint two vertical stripes on your nail.

Using the striping brush and black polish or acrylic paint, create short lines angling up from the sidewall to the first vertical stripe.

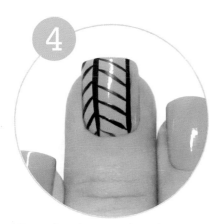

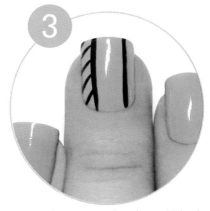

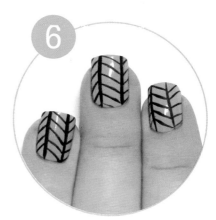

Paint short lines angling down between the two vertical lines.

Paint a final set of short lines, this time angled upwards, between the second vertical line and other sidewall.

Finish your manicure by repeating steps 2 through 5 on all of your nails.

Foil Accents

Nail foils can add a glitzy finish to a classic manicure. This technique requires no special tools aside from the nail foils, which are available in many colours and designs. (Cut them to fit and have them ready before you paint your nails.) Here, red foil and red polish create a glowing monochromatic look.

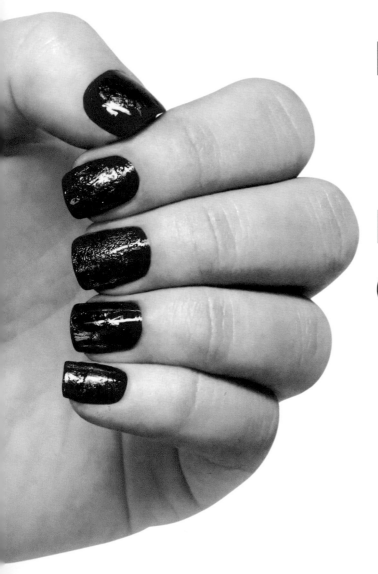

MATERIALS

Scissors

Red nail foils

Top coat

POLISH COLOURS

Red

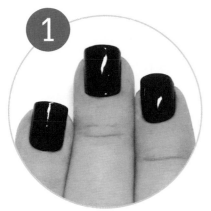

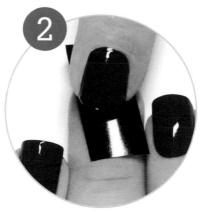

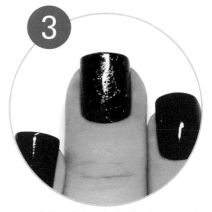

Polish your nails red. Let them dry until still just slightly sticky.

Take a pre-cut piece of nail foil and gently press it on your sticky nail.

Carefully lift the foil off of the nail, leaving some of the shiny foil behind. This technique creates a textured marbled look.

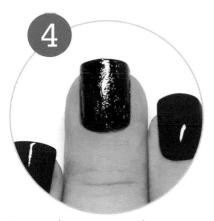

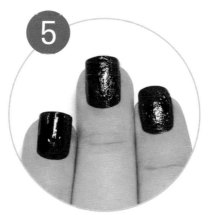

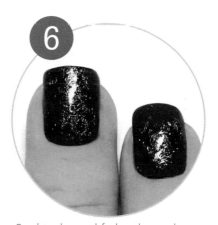

Repeat this process until you are pleased with the effect on your nail.

Repeat steps 2 through 4 on each nail. If the polish dries, apply top coat, let dry until just sticky, and proceed.

Seal in the nail foil with two layers of top coat.

Rhinestone Accents

Nothing flashes more brightly than rhinestones and crystals, especially on your nails. By using a variety of differently coloured rhinestones in a range of sizes and shapes, you can create a texturally interesting manicure that looks complex but actually requires little effort.

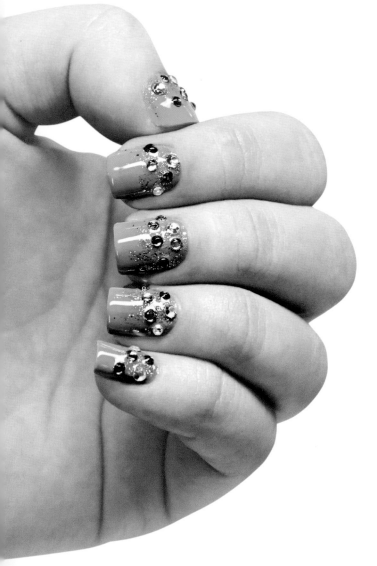

MATERIALS

Top coat (not quick-dry)   Tweezers

Nail glue (optional)   Rhinestones

POLISH COLOURS

Blue   Silver glitter

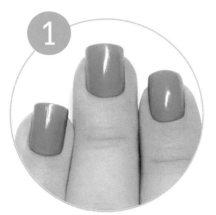

Polish your nails blue. Let them dry for a few minutes.

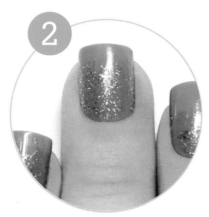

Polish each nail with a splash of silver glitter polish, starting from the cuticle to about two-thirds up the nail.

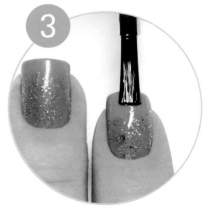

Apply a layer of top coat to one nail. For a stronger hold, use nail glue instead.

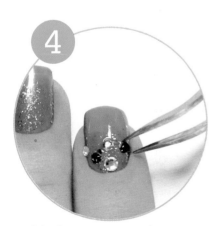

While the top coat or glue is wet, use tweezers to apply a variety of rhinestones over the glitter polish.

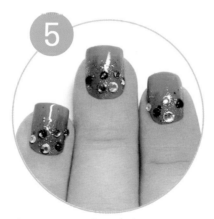

Repeat steps 3 and 4 on your other nails. Add stones until you are happy with the effect.

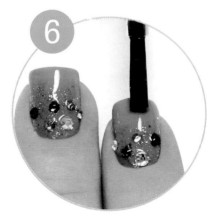

Once dry, carefully apply a thick layer of top coat over the stones.

Floating Heart

Hearts, which can be created simply using a dotting tool and a striping brush, will become a crucial part of your nail art skill set. In this manicure, romantic colours come together for a perfect Valentine's Day look.

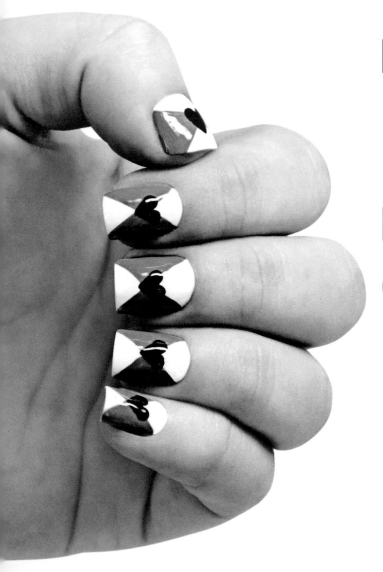

MATERIALS

Striping brush

Dotting tool

Polish palette

POLISH COLOURS

White   Pink   Red

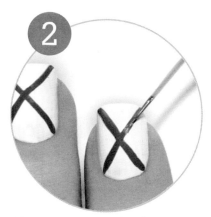

Polish your nails white. Let them dry for a few minutes.

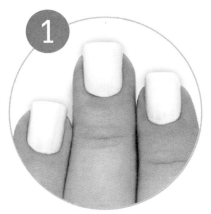

Using your striping brush, paint a pink 'X' on each nail.

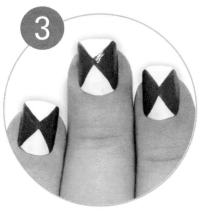

Using your striping brush, fill in the sides of the 'X' with pink polish. Let your nails dry briefly.

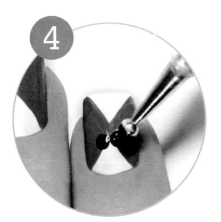

To create the heart, use your dotting tool to make two red dots close together in the centre of one nail.

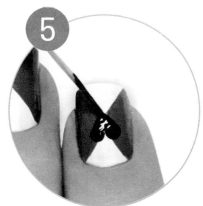

Use your striping brush loaded with red polish to gently pull the dots down into a point, to create a heart.

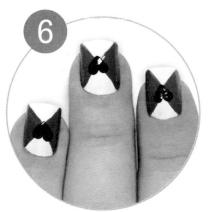

Complete steps 4 and 5 on each nail.

Chequerboards

Bold black-and-white chequerboard nails are perfect for a weekend of Grand Prix motor racing. Pair a chequerboard accent nail with a bright neon manicure for a lively contrasting look.

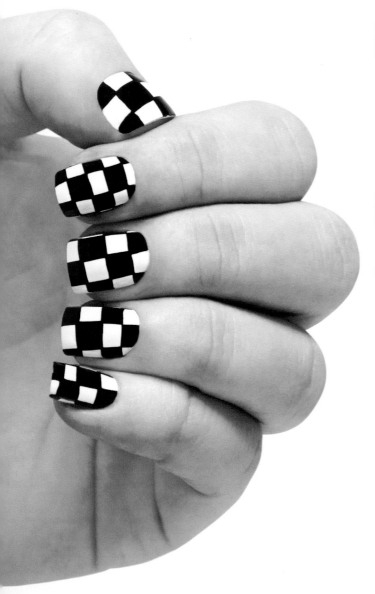

POLISH COLOURS

 White Black

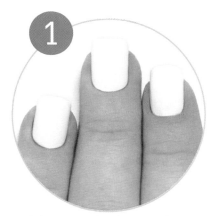

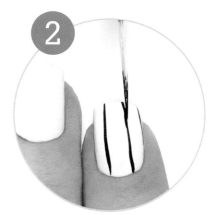

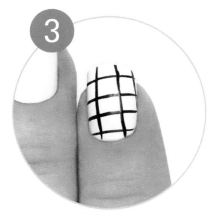

Polish your nails white. Let them dry for a few minutes.

Using your striping brush and black polish or acrylic paint, create two or three evenly spaced vertical lines on your nail.

In a similar fashion, create horizontal lines, making a grid of squares on the nail.

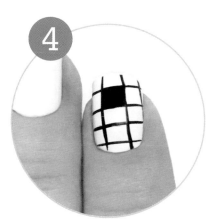

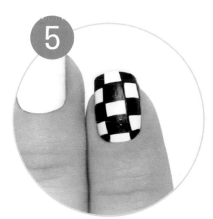

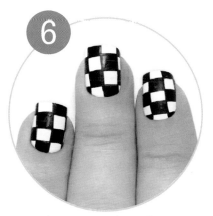

Using the tip of your striping brush, fill paint one square in the grid black.

Continue out from the black square, completing the grid in a chequerboard pattern.

Complete steps 2 through 5 on the rest of your nails, or wear the chequerboard design as an accent nail. Add a top coat to complete the look.

Vertical Line

This design uses striping tape to enable you to contrast white with two of your favourite polish shades in one manicure. Choose bold, contrasting shades for a wild and attention-grabbing look, or several shades of polish from the same colour family for a more subtle finish.

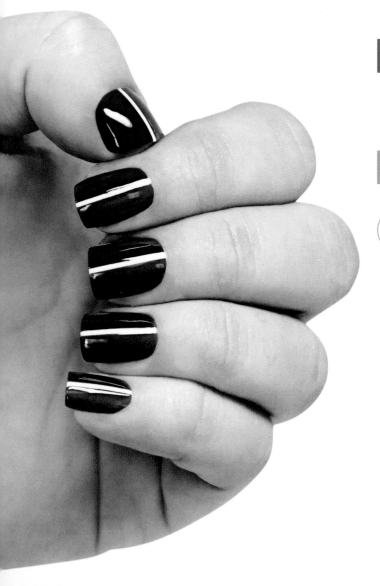

MATERIALS

Striping tape

POLISH COLOURS

White   Blue   Purple

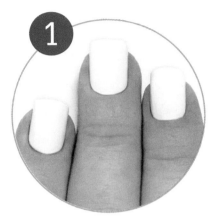

Polish your nails white. Let them dry for a few minutes.

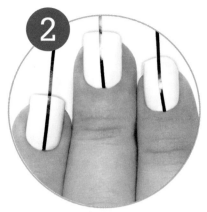

Apply a single piece of striping tape down the centre of each nail.

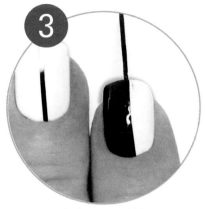

Polish half of one nail blue, being careful not to cross over the striping tape.

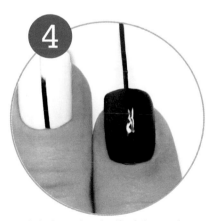

Polish the other half of the nail purple, once again being careful not to paint over the tape.

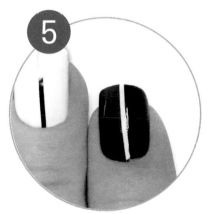

Straight after polishing, remove the striping tape. If the polish dries before you remove it, the line will not be as sharp.

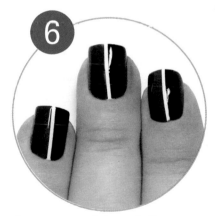

Repeat steps 3 through 5 on the rest of your nails.

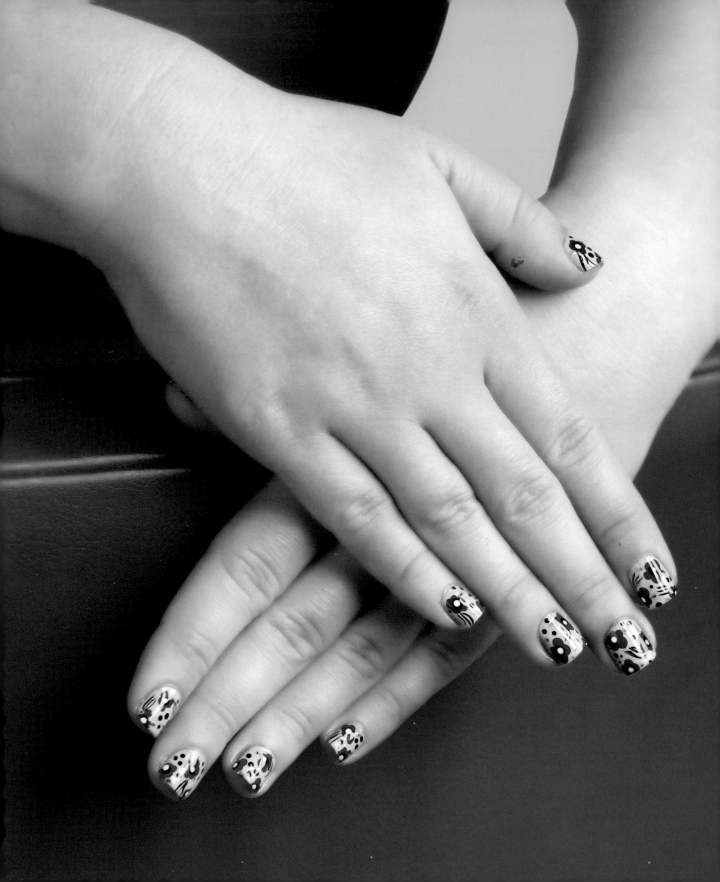

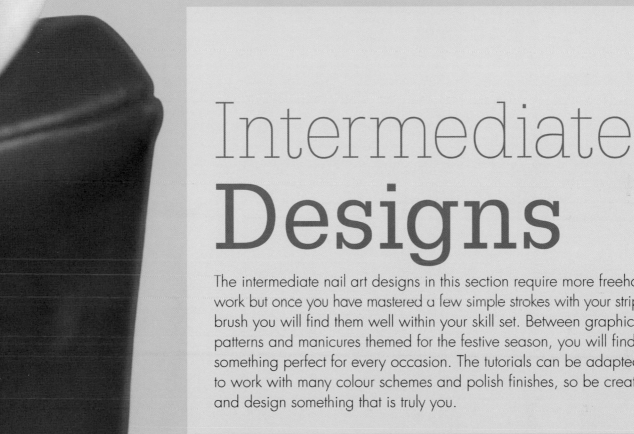

Intermediate
Designs

The intermediate nail art designs in this section require more freehand work but once you have mastered a few simple strokes with your striping brush you will find them well within your skill set. Between graphic patterns and manicures themed for the festive season, you will find something perfect for every occasion. The tutorials can be adapted to work with many colour schemes and polish finishes, so be creative and design something that is truly you.

Black Tie

When you attend a formal affair, your nails need to look the part as well. Adorn your nails in their own black tie and you will have a conversation starter at your fingertips.

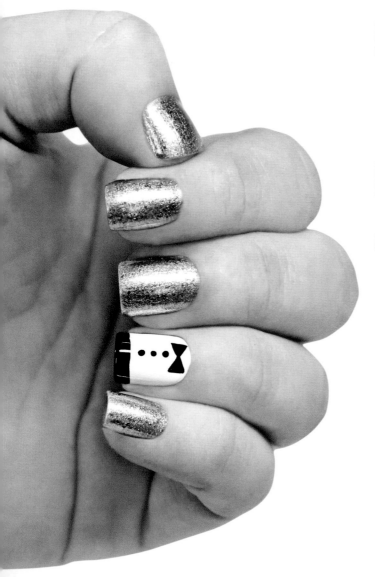

MATERIALS	
Tape	Dotting tool
Striping brush	Polish palette

POLISH COLOURS

Gold   White   Black

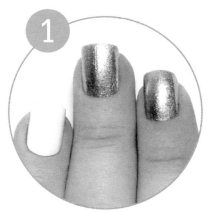

Polish your nails gold with a white accent nail. Let them dry for a few minutes.

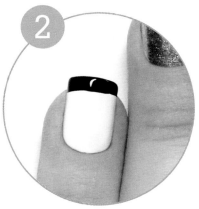

Paint a black French tip on the white nail. Use tape for this if it's easier for you.

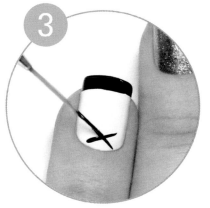

Near the base of your nail, paint an 'X' shape in black polish or acrylic paint with your striping brush.

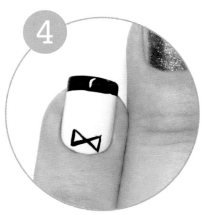

Paint two small lines to close off the 'X' into a black-tie shape.

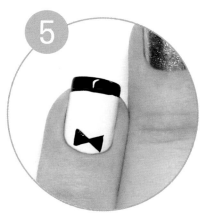

Using your striping brush, carefully fill tie outline with black paint.

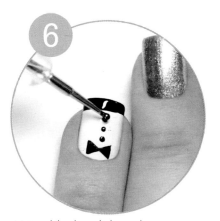

Using black polish and your dotting tool, create two or three 'buttons' down the centre of the nail.

Sunburst

By combining both sponging and striping-tape techniques, you can create a wide variety of bold graphic looks. In this manicure, the tape is lifted to reveal a gradation of summertime colours that really pop against the black polish.

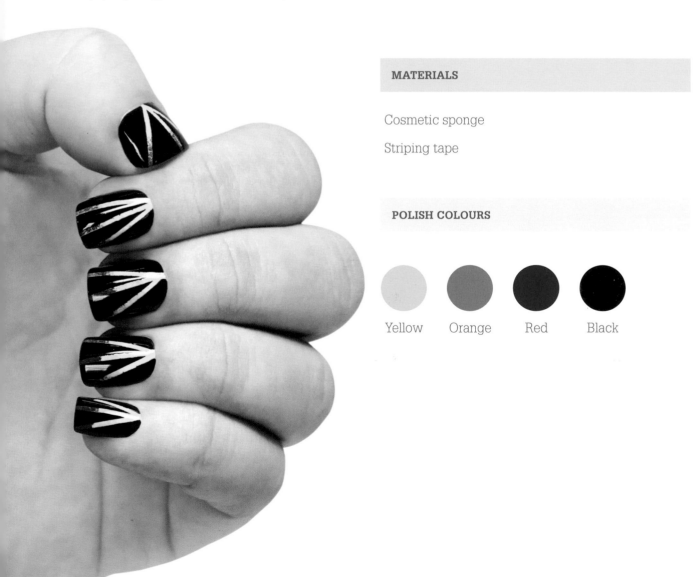

MATERIALS

Cosmetic sponge

Striping tape

POLISH COLOURS

Yellow   Orange   Red   Black

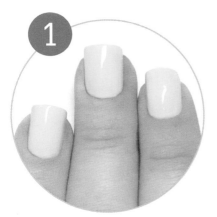

Polish your nails yellow. Let them dry for a few minutes.

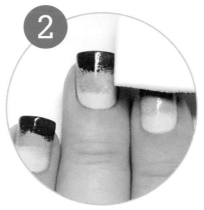

Use a cosmetic sponge to apply orange polish to the half of your nail closest to the free edge and red polish to the very tip of each nail. Let them dry for a few minutes.

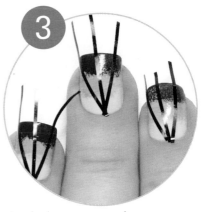

Apply three pieces of striping tape to each nail, in a fan shape, starting at the cuticle.

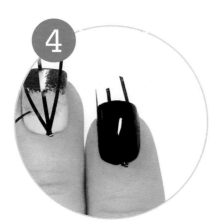

Polish all over the nail plate and striping tape with black polish on one nail.

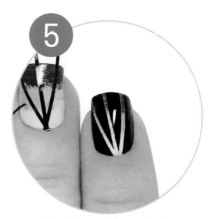

Straight after polishing (before it dries), carefully remove the striping tape to reveal the colour beneath.

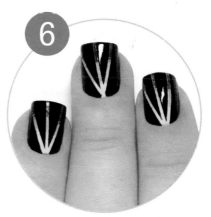

Repeat steps 4 and 5 on the rest of your nails.

Tree Nail

Whatever the season, trees are always an imaginative motif. This tutorial shows you how to create a basic tree, but as you become more adept at using your striping brush, you can create larger trees with more branches.

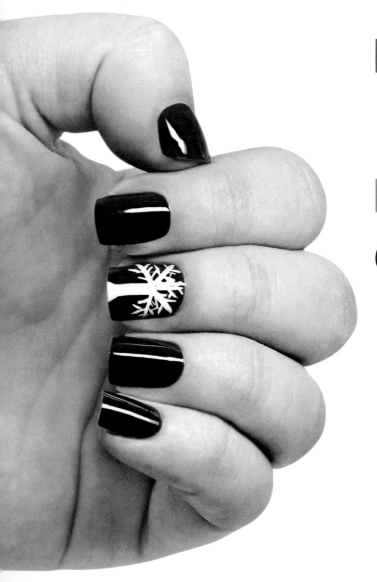

MATERIALS

Striping brush

Polish palette

POLISH COLOURS

Dark green White

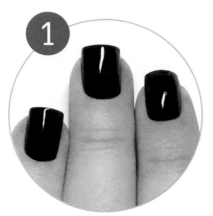

Polish your nails dark green. Let them dry for a few minutes.

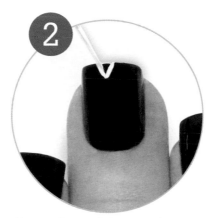

Using white polish or acrylic paint and your striping brush, paint a small triangle at the tip of your nail.

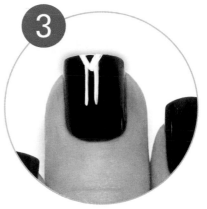

Paint two vertical lines coming down from the small triangle, creating the 'trunk' of the tree.

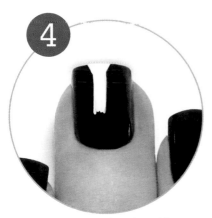

Use your striping brush to fill in the tree trunk.

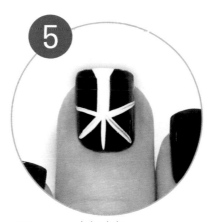

Paint several thick lines coming out of the trunk. These are the main branches.

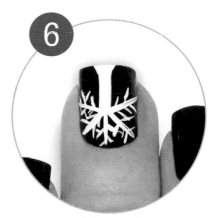

Paint several thinner, shorter lines off of each thicker branch, completing the tree.

Glitter Heart

Heart manicures are a favourite for Valentine's Day or any time you want to celebrate romance. This manicure combines soft, feminine shades with sparkling glitter, a contrast that is always stylish.

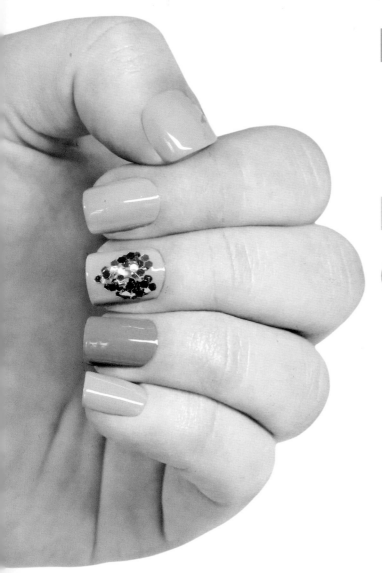

Top coat (not quick-dry)

Dotting tool

Pink hexagonal glitter sequins

POLISH COLOURS

Grey   Pink

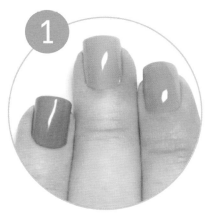

Paint your nails grey with a pink accent nail on your ring finger nail. Let them dry for a few minutes.

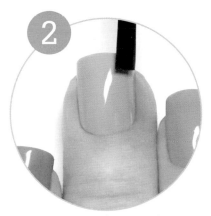

On your middle finger nail, apply a layer of top coat.

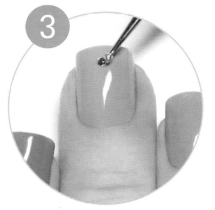

Using a dotting tool dipped in top coat, place a pink glitter sequin on to the middle finger nail, centred near the free edge.

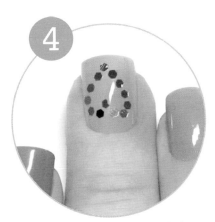

Continue placing individual glitter sequins on your nail, creating the outline of a heart.

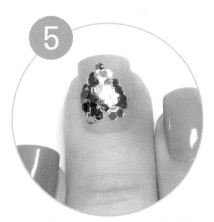

Use glitter sequins to completely fill the heart shape.

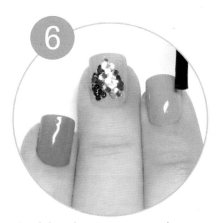

Seal the glitter sequins in place with two layers of top coat.

Snowflake

Whether you live in a cold climate or somewhere tropical, snowflake nail art always brings a unique elegance. This manicure features one subtle snowflake, but you could also create a blizzard of flakes on all ten nails.

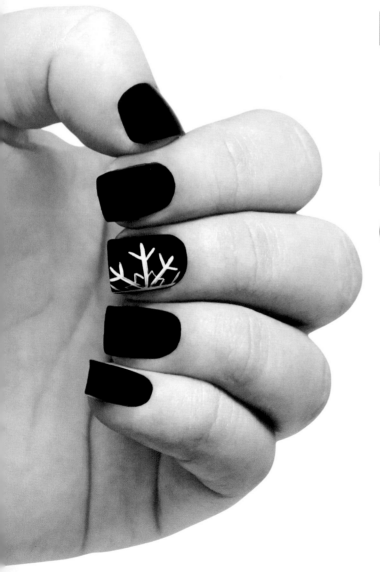

MATERIALS

Polish palette

Striping brush

POLISH COLOURS

Dark
purple

White

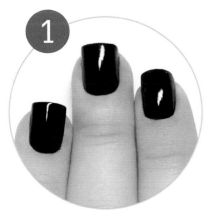

Polish your nails dark purple. Let them dry for a few minutes.

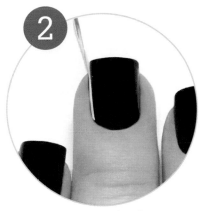

Using your striping brush and white polish or acrylic paint, paint one vertical line against the sidewall on your accent nail.

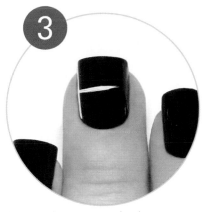

Paint a line perpendicular to the vertical line you created in step 2.

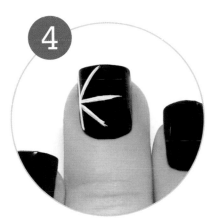

Paint two more lines diagonally out from the sidewall, creating the rays of the snowflake.

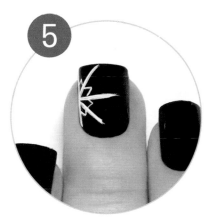

Using the striping brush, carefully create small V-shapes between each ray of the snowflake.

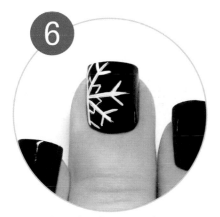

Complete the design with small lines coming off of each ray of the snowflake.

Boho Floral

This funky floral pattern is created with nothing more complicated than dots and a few simple strokes using your striping brush. Once it's complete, you'll be ready for the beach or a summer music festival. Combine bold, contrasting shades for an eye-catching look.

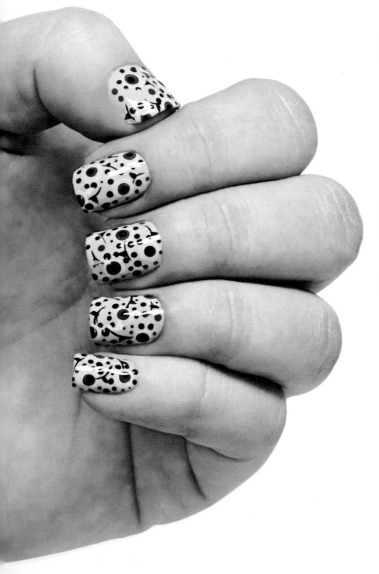

MATERIALS

Dotting tool

Polish palette

Striping brush

POLISH COLOURS

| Beige | Light blue | Coral | Purple | Black |

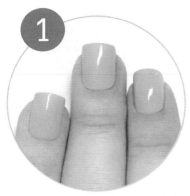

Paint your nails in beige polish. Let them dry for a few minutes.

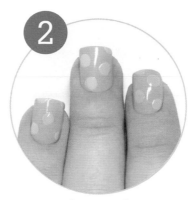

Use your dotting tool to create large light blue dots spaced evenly across your nails.

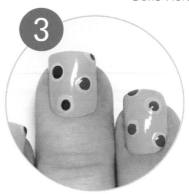

Clean your dotting tool and then use it to place a dot of coral polish in the centre of each blue dot.

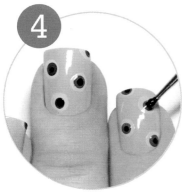

Use the smaller end of your dotting tool to place tiny purple dots in the centre of each coral dot. These are your flowers.

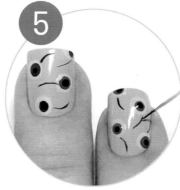

Using your striping brush and black polish or acrylic paint, paint small curved lines extending from each flower.

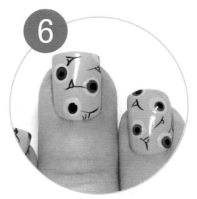

Using your striping brush again, paint a small triangle 'leaf' coming from each stem.

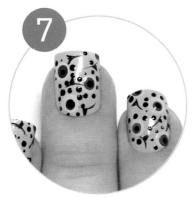

Carefully fill in each triangle-shaped leaf with black polish or acrylic paint.

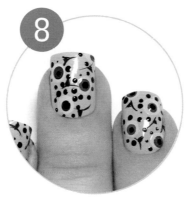

Using your dotting tool and black polish, place small black dots around each flower shape.

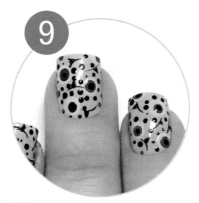

Fill in any empty space on the nail with tiny coral dots.

Ikat

Nails painted with graphic patterns work well for most occasions and all ages. This design, inspired by ikat textile patterns, is easy to create as none of the lines are precise. You can use any combination of polish colours you like to match your outfit or your mood.

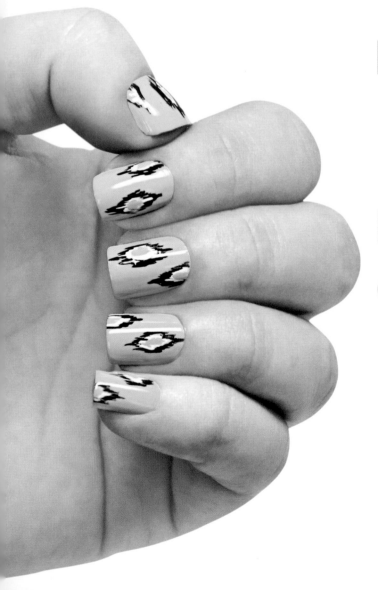

MATERIALS

Striping brush

Polish palette

Top coat

POLISH COLOURS

Blue   Black   White

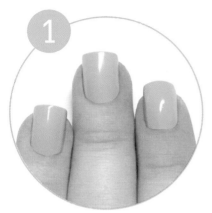

Polish your nails blue. Let them dry for a few minutes.

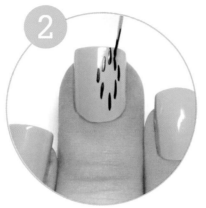

Using a striping brush and black polish or acrylic paint, paint a series of short, black, vertical lines on one nail, outlining a diamond shape.

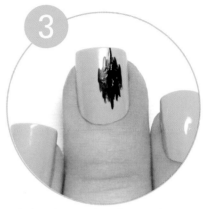

Fill the diamond outline with more vertical black lines, creating a more solid diamond shape.

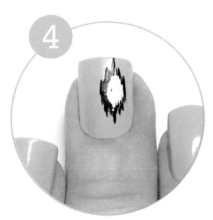

Using white polish or acrylic paint and your striping brush, paint a similar smaller white diamond shape within the black one.

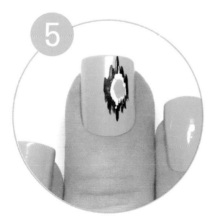

Use your striping brush to add a small blue diamond in the centre of the white diamond.

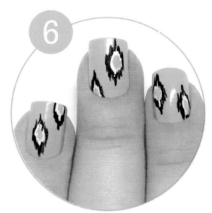

Repeat steps 2 through 5, spacing out the pattern across all of your nails. Add a layer of top coat to complete the look.

Tropical Floral

Tropical floral designs are perfect for manicures and pedicures when you are in a Caribbean holiday frame of mind. This tutorial shows how to create an all-over floral print, but you could easily paint just one flower at the base of each nail (or toenail) for a chic effect.

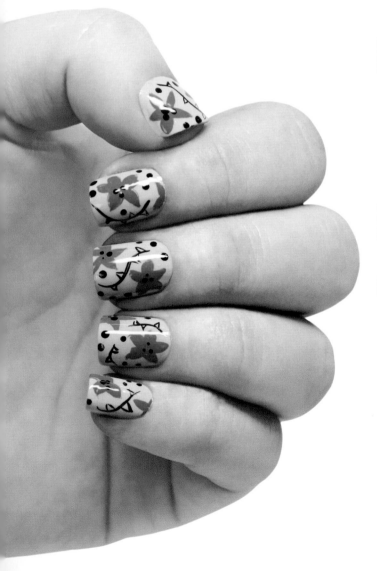

MATERIALS

Striping brush

Polish palette

Dotting tool

POLISH COLOURS

Beige   Pink   Black

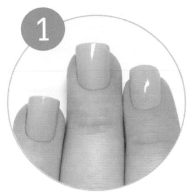

Polish your nails a beige shade.

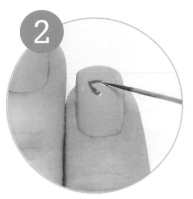

Using your striping brush loaded with pink polish, paint two curved brushstrokes that meet at a point.

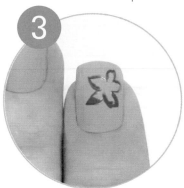

Repeat step 2, creating a flower shape with five petals. You can also make four-point flowers.

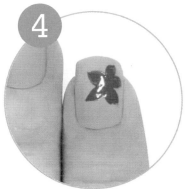

Use your striping brush to fill up the flower shape with pink polish.

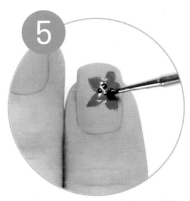

Using your dotting tool and black polish, create three small dots in the centre of the flower.

Repeat steps 2 through 5, filling your nails with flowers. For a complete look, create some partial flowers at the edges of your nails.

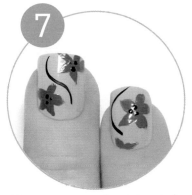

Use your striping brush loaded with black polish or acrylic paint to create curved lines between the flowers.

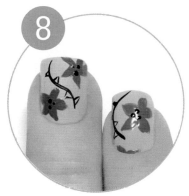

Use your striping brush to carefully add triangle-shaped leaves to the lines.

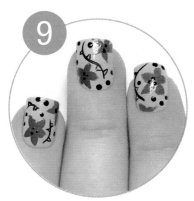

Using your dotting tool and black polish, fill any empty space on your nails with small dots.

Easter Egg

In the springtime, pastel egg motifs are everywhere. This delightful design makes a great accent nail paired with polka dots in many sizes.

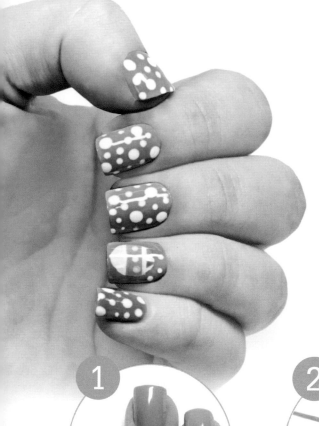

MATERIALS	
Striping brush	Dotting tool
Polish palette	Top coat

POLISH COLOURS

Pastel yellow   Pastel pink   Pastel purple   Orange   White

1

Polish your nails orange with a pastel yellow accent nail. The pastel nail will be your Easter egg nail.

2

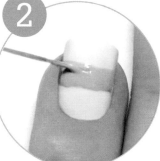

On your accent nail, use your striping brush and pastel pink polish to create a horizontal stripe in the centre of your nail.

3

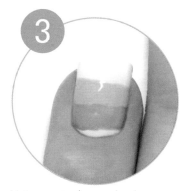

Using a similar method, paint a pastel purple horizontal stripe below the pink one you just created.

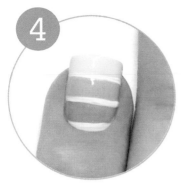

Load your striping brush with white polish or acrylic paint and make straight lines above and below the pastel stripes where they meet.

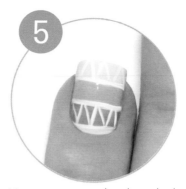

Use your striping brush and white polish or acrylic paint to create tiny zigzags on the yellow and purple stripes.

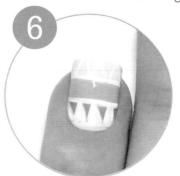

Carefully fill in the staggered triangles you just created within the zigzags on the purple stripe.

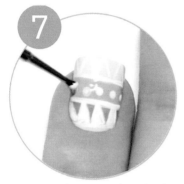

Use your dotting tool and white polish to create small dots on the pink stripe.

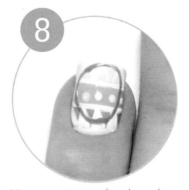

Use your striping brush and orange polish to carefully outline the shape of an egg over the pastel design you just created.

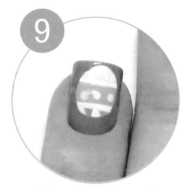

Carefully paint the rest of the nail with orange polish, revealing an egg shape in the centre filled with pretty designs.

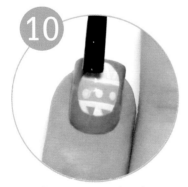

Paint the accent nail with a top coat to smooth out the patterned design.

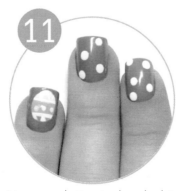

Use your dotting tool and white polish to create several large dots, spaced randomly across the nails you painted orange.

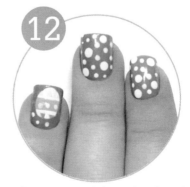

Fill any space left on the dotted orange nails using the small end of your dotting tool and white polish.

Geometric Manicure

Graphical geometric manicures are right on trend. This tutorial suggests several patterns that work well together, but feel free to experiment with your own ideas. Once you have chosen your pattern, you could even pair it with a textural or gradient background for an impressive manicure.

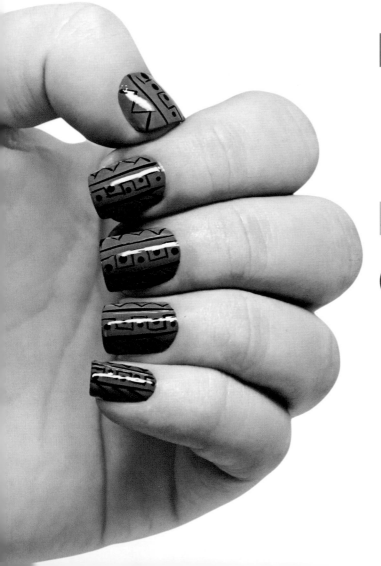

MATERIALS

Striping brush

Polish palette

Dotting tool

POLISH COLOURS

Pink   Black

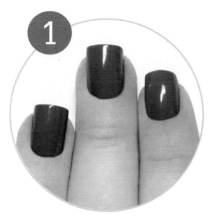

Polish your nails pink. Let them dry for a few minutes.

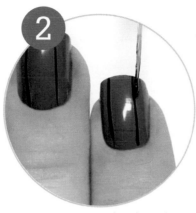

Using your striping brush and black polish or acrylic paint, create two vertical lines on each nail.

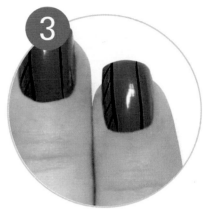

Using your striping brush again, paint short lines slanting upwards between the sidewall and the first vertical line.

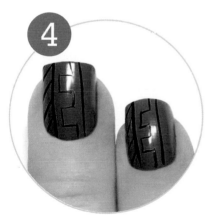

Between the two vertical lines, carefully paint small line segments, creating the geometric pattern shown.

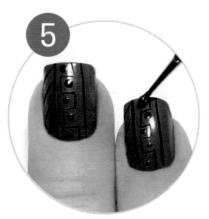

Using your dotting tool and black polish, place a small dot in each notch of the design you just made.

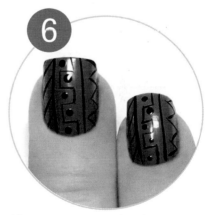

Using your striping brush, create a zigzag line between the second vertical line and the sidewall.

V-Gaps

Can't decide which of your two favourite polishes to wear? Use them both in this intriguing design. Simple lines and dots in contrasting colours virtually pop off the nail. For a subtler look, skip the polka dots or use polishes of the same hue.

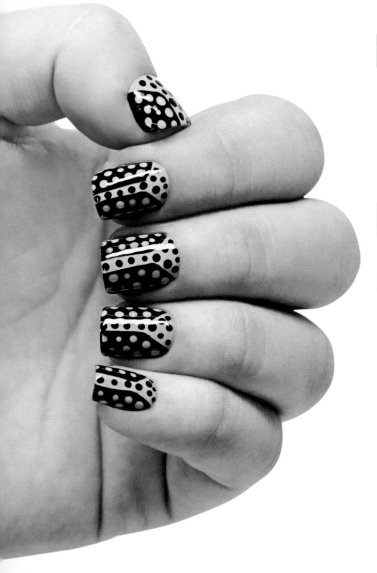

MATERIALS

Striping brush

Polish palette

Dotting tool

POLISH COLOURS

Grey   Dark
        purple

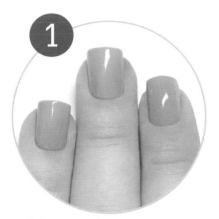

Polish your nails grey. Let them dry for a few minutes.

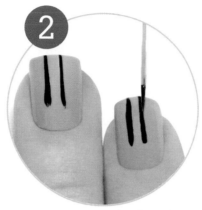

Using your striping brush and dark purple polish, paint two vertical lines from the tip of your nail that stop about two thirds of the way down.

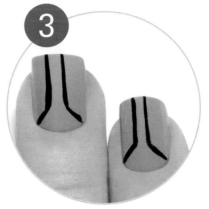

Paint two more lines at an angle from the first ones, connecting to the corner of your nail near the cuticle.

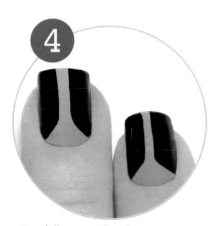

Carefully paint the shapes you just created near the sidewalls in dark purple, leaving the grey centre exposed.

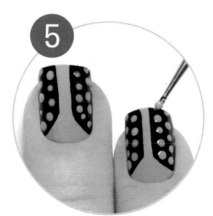

Using your dotting tool, fill the dark purple areas with small grey dots.

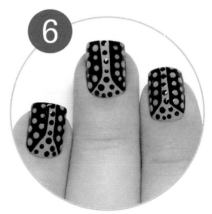

Again using your dotting tool, fill the grey area with small dark purple dots.

Splash Floral

Bright and spring-like, the Splash Floral manicure is perfect for warm weather or those who want to start with subtle nail art. This manicure uses a bright yellow colour scheme, but pink, purple, or lime green would work wonderfully as well.

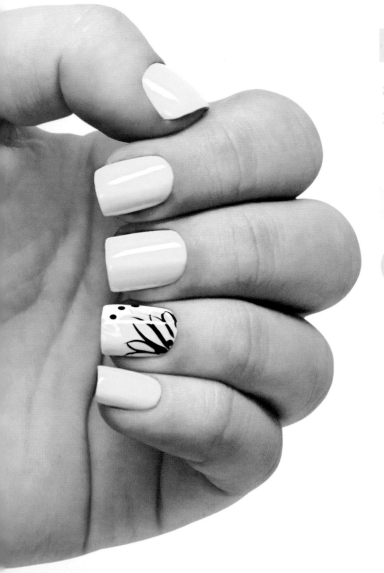

MATERIALS	
Striping brush	Dotting tool
Polish palette	Kitchen paper

POLISH COLOURS

Yellow   White   Black

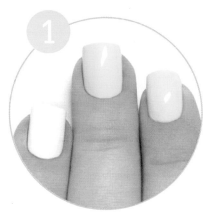

Polish your nails yellow with a white accent nail. Let them dry for a few minutes.

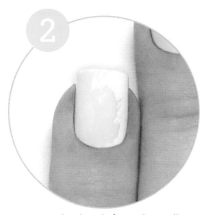

Remove the brush from the yellow polish bottle and wipe most of the polish off of it on to some kitchen paper. On the white nail, use the dry brush to create a splash of color coming up from the cuticle.

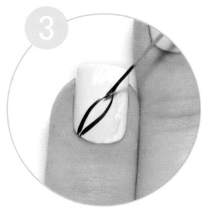

Using your striping brush and black polish or acrylic paint, create a petal shape over the yellow splash. Flowing strokes work best.

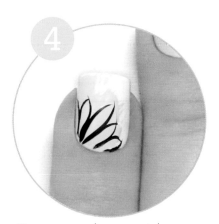

Create several more petals, filling the corner of your nail.

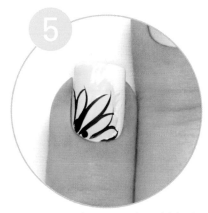

Using your dotting tool and black polish, create two or three small dots in the centre of the flower.

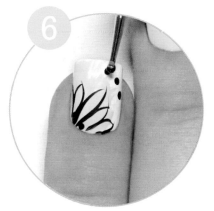

To create some movement on the nail, add three small dots in a curved shape towards the tip of the nail.

Hydrangeas

What flower could be more captivating or feminine than a blue hydrangea? This technique combines several shades of blue to create the iconic blooms using simple polka dots. When paired with a soft pink, this manicure is perfect for a wedding in early spring.

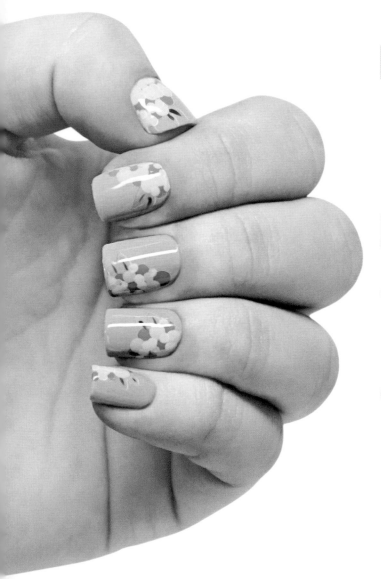

MATERIALS

Dotting tool

Polish palette

Striping brush

POLISH COLOURS

Soft pink

True blue

Light green

Dark green

Light blue

Medium blue

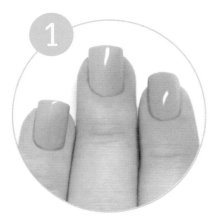

Polish your nails soft pink. Let them dry for a few minutes.

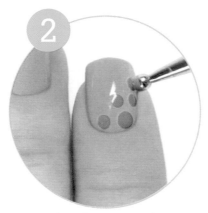

On each nail, create a cluster of true blue dots. You can place them in different spots on each nail.

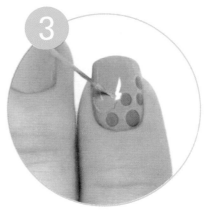

Using your striping brush and a light green polish, paint two triangular leaves coming off of each cluster of blue dots.

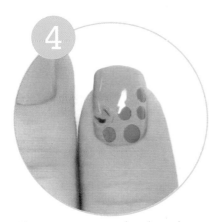

Using your striping brush and dark green polish, add an accent line down the centre of each leaf.

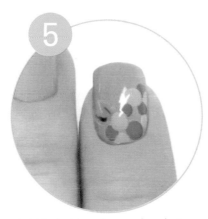

Add light blue dots to the cluster you started in step 2, covering the edges of the leaves.

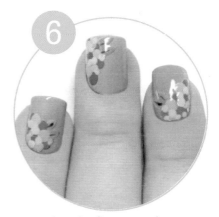

Complete the flowers with more dots in a medium blue shade, being sure to cover most of the pink polish within the flower.

Poppy Floral

This all-over floral pattern features autumnal colours, but you could wear this design any time of year. Fanciful details and dots in this manicure make it original and eye-catching.

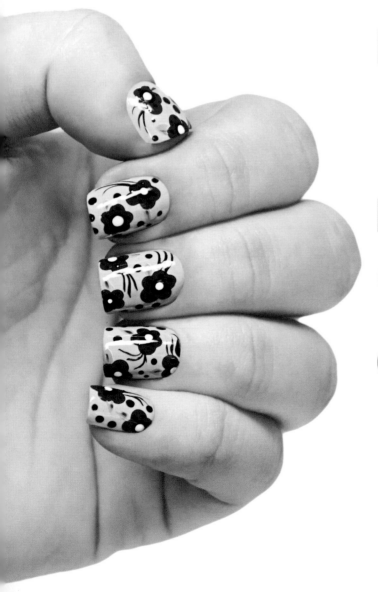

Dotting tool

Polish palette

Striping brush

POLISH COLOURS

Beige

Red

Black

White

Light green

Dark green

Brown

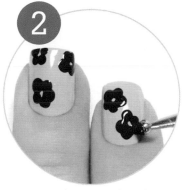

1

Polish your nails in a beige shade. Let them dry for a few minutes.

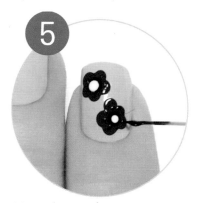

2

Use your dotting tool and red polish to create five dots connected in a circular fashion. Space them over your nails.

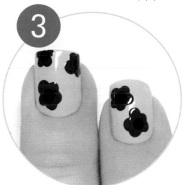

3

Use your dotting tool and black polish to add a black dot in the centre of each flower.

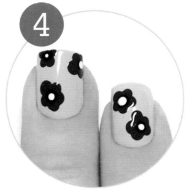

4

Use the small end of your dotting tool and white polish to add a small white dot to the centre of each flower.

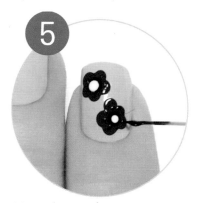

5

Using the tip of your striping brush and black polish, encircle the black centre of each flower with tiny black dots.

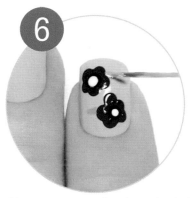

6

Use your striping brush and a light green polish to create triangular leaves extending from each flower.

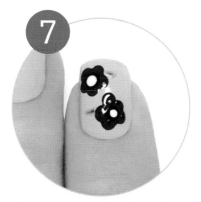

7

Use your striping brush and a dark green polish to add an accent line down the centre of each leaf.

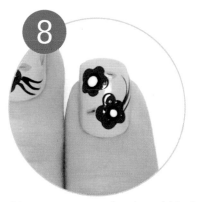

8

Using your striping brush and black polish, create short, curved lines coming from a few of the flowers.

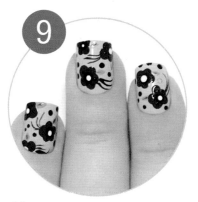

9

Fill any empty space on your nails with small, brown dots.

Wood Grain

The nature lover in all of us can enjoy this simple nail pattern. No two trees are the same, so each nail can be slightly different and imperfect. Let your creativity flow as you make the smooth brushstrokes in this design.

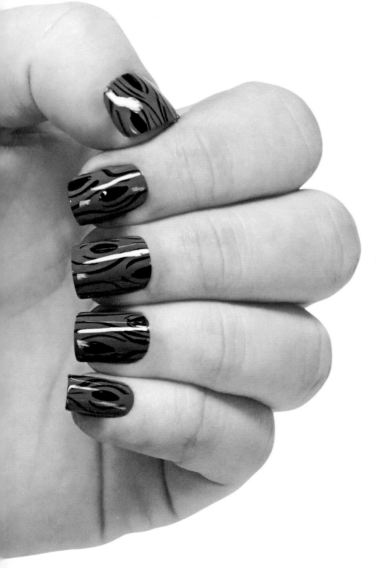

MATERIALS

Polish palette

Striping brush

POLISH COLOURS

Brown   Black

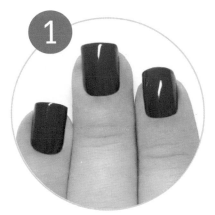

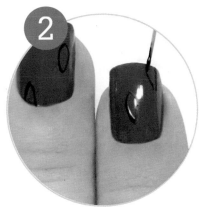

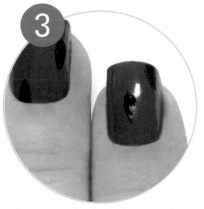

Polish your nails brown. Let them dry for a few minutes.

Using your striping brush and black polish or acrylic paint, paint one or two rugby ball shapes on each nail.

Fill each rugby ball shape with black polish or acrylic paint.

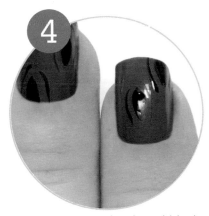

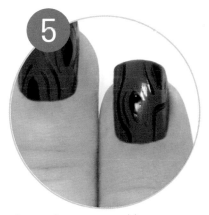

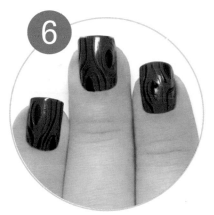

Use your striping brush and black polish or acrylic paint to create short, curved lines round the long sides of each rugby ball shape.

Create longer curved lines that go around the shorter curved lines.

Finish the wood grain with a few more curved lines to fill the nail.

Spiderwebs

Hallowe'en is the perfect time to dress up your finger nails. Spiderwebs are a great seasonal motif and are simple to create using straight and curved lines. Orange and black contrast well, but you can also try using different colour combinations on each nail for a festive look.

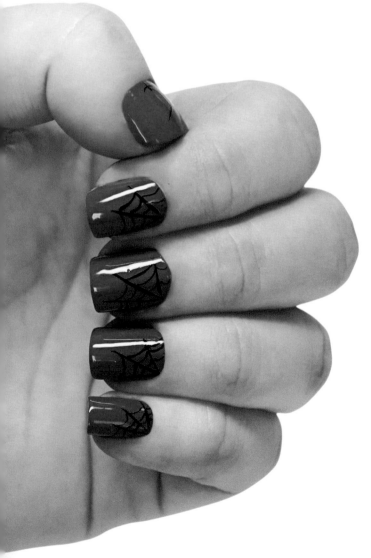

MATERIALS

Polish palette

Striping brush

POLISH COLOURS

Orange   Black

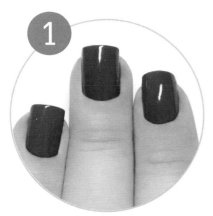

Polish your nails orange. Let them dry for a few minutes.

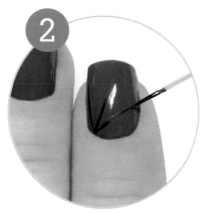

Use your striping brush and black polish or acrylic paint to create three lines at the base of your nail, extending out from the corner.

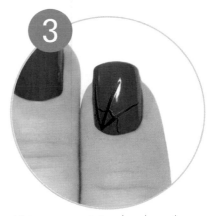

Using your striping brush and black polish or paint, create a small U-shape between each of the lines you made in step 2.

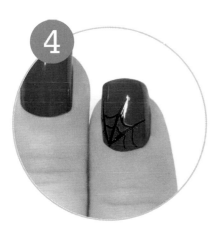

Repeat step 3, moving closer to the ends of the lines. Your U-shapes will be larger than in step 3.

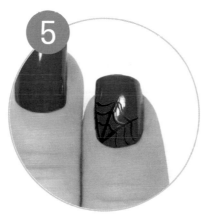

Again, repeat the technique, creating a larger U-shape between each line. Repeat as needed until your web is complete.

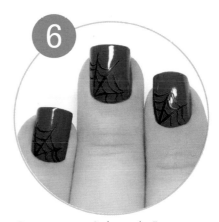

Repeat steps 2 through 5 on all nails, or wear the spiderweb as an accent nail.

Baroque Vines

Abstract vines are a great alternative to floral nails. When done in a navy colour scheme, they are reminiscent of fine china. The techniques in this manicure are simple, but you have a lot of creative control in the placement of the vines.

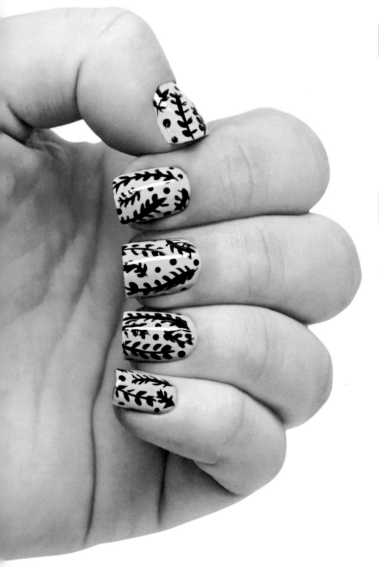

Beige   Navy

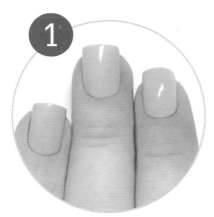

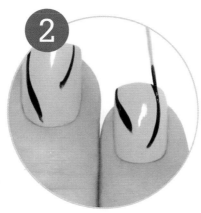

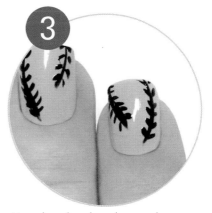

Polish your nails beige. Let them dry for a few minutes.

Using your striping brush loaded with navy polish, create one or two long, curved lines on each nail.

Use short brushstrokes and navy polish to create leaf shapes extending from the lines you created in step 2.

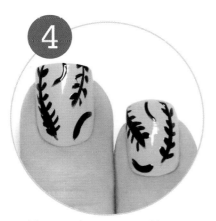

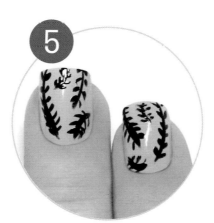

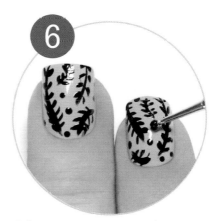

Add some shorter curved lines where there is space on the nail.

As in step 3, create leaf shapes on the shorter lines.

Fill any empty space on the nail with small navy dots.

Gingerbread Nails

This witty manicure turns your nails into an clever version of a traditional Christmas gingerbread cookie. White polish acts as the icing, creating a unique manicure that is sure to get attention.

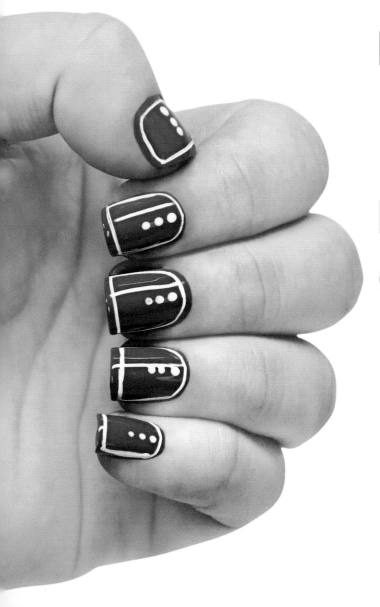

MATERIALS

Striping brush

Polish palette

Dotting tool

POLISH COLOURS

Brown   White

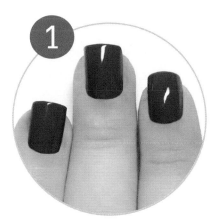

Polish your nails in a brown polish. Let them dry for a few minutes.

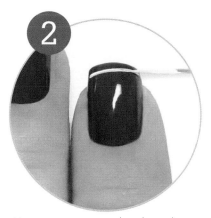

Using your striping brush and white polish or acrylic paint, create a line along the free edge of one nail. Follow the shape of your natural nail.

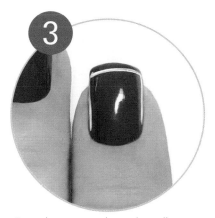

Paint lines near the sidewall on each side of your nail, again following the shape of your nail bed.

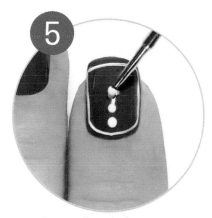

Finish the outline of your nail by following the curve of your cuticle.

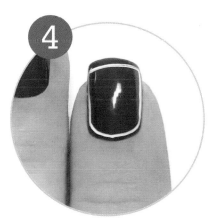

Use the small end of your dotting tool and white polish to create two or three dots from the cuticle, up the centre of the nail.

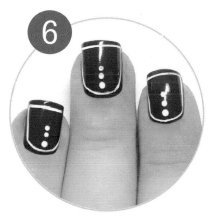

Complete steps 2 through 5 on your other nails. If desired, paint a final line beside the 'buttons', as seen in the main image.

Tweed

Textural manicures are striking and highly fashionable. In this manicure, shades of black and white are layered to create a textile-like finish that goes with anything.

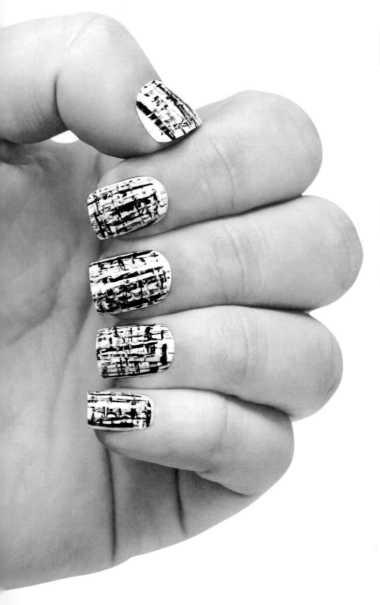

MATERIALS

Striping brush

Polish palette

Kitchen paper

POLISH COLOURS

White   Black   Grey

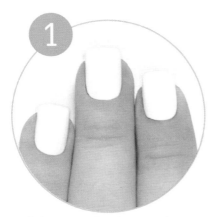

Polish your nails white. Let them dry for a few minutes.

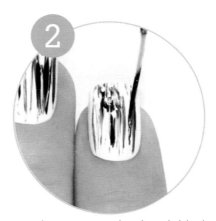

Load your striping brush with black polish and wipe it off on some kitchen paper, leaving only a small amount of polish on the bristles. Create several vertical brushstrokes on the nail.

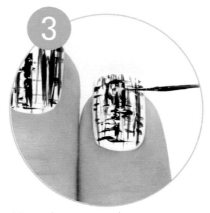

Using the same technique, create horizontal strokes across the nail in black.

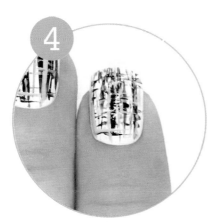

Layer a series of vertical and horizontal grey brushstrokes over the black ones.

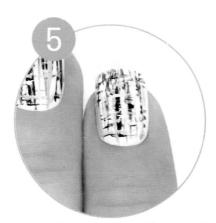

Layer white vertical and horizontal brushstrokes over the entire nail.

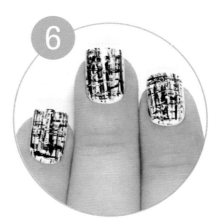

If needed, go back in with several more black brushstrokes to create more depth on the nail.

Tape Tree

Using clear adhesive tape and striping tape, you can create a crisp Christmas tree manicure without using any freehand art. Pair it with polka dots and festive colours for a captivating seasonal look.

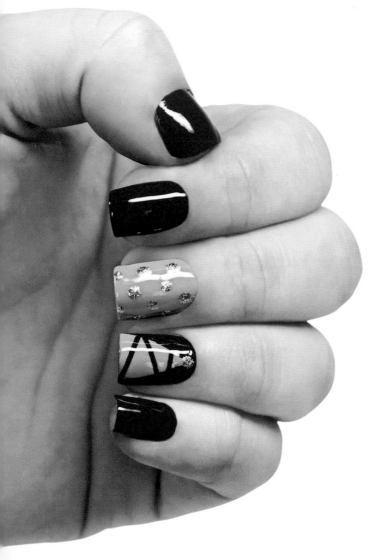

MATERIALS

Clear adhesive tape

Striping tape

Dotting tool

Polish palette

POLISH COLOURS

Red   Green   Gold

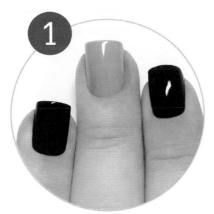

Paint your nails red with a green accent nail on your middle finger. Let them dry completely.

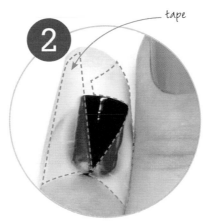

On the ring finger nail, apply two pieces of tape that come to a point near the base of the nail, leaving a triangle shape exposed.

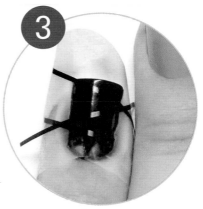

Add three or four pieces of striping tape in a zigzag pattern over the exposed nail.

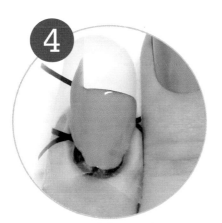

Paint green polish over the exposed part of the nail.

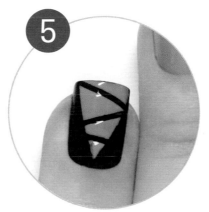

Immediately after applying polish, carefully remove both types of tape.

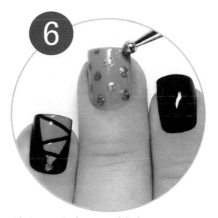

If desired, fix a gold dot to the tip of the tree you just created and more gold dots on the green accent nail.

Art Deco Tips

Artistic black-and-white nails are a classic any time of year. If you are very patient, you could use striping tape to re-create this eclectic French visual arts style, but here is how to create a clean, structural look using your striping brush.

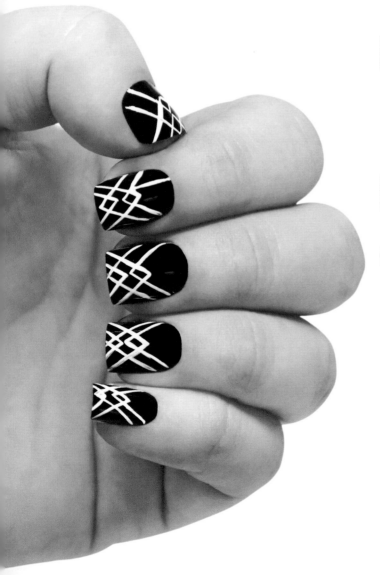

MATERIALS

Striping brush

Polish palette

POLISH COLOURS

Black　　White

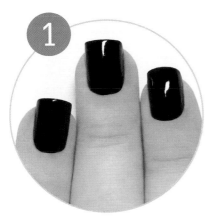

Polish your nails black. Let them dry for a few minutes.

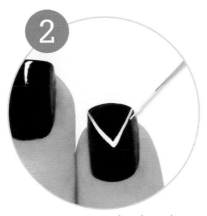

Using your striping brush and white polish or acrylic paint, paint a V-shape on one nail, starting at the free edge and coming to a point in the centre of the nail.

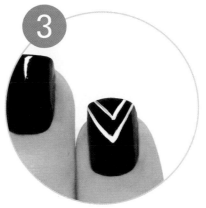

Using the same technique, paint a smaller V-shape within the first one.

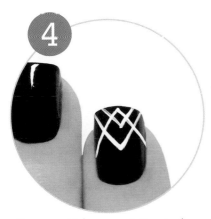

Create a V-shape pointing in the opposite direction, coming to a point within the V from step 3.

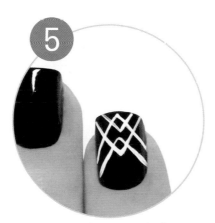

Repeat step 4, starting farther down the nail.

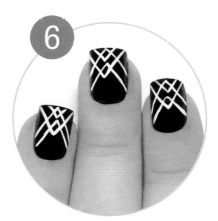

Repeat steps 2 through 5 on the rest of your nails.

Chevrons

Vividly coloured chevrons are perfect for a summertime manicure. This design uses striping tape to create crisp white lines that contrast nicely against the bright colours. You can also use the chevron design as an accent nail to add interest to your manicure.

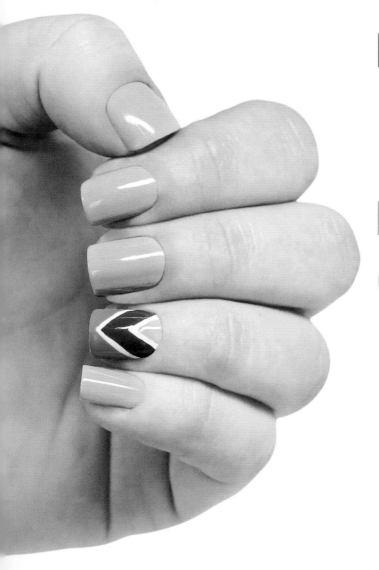

MATERIALS

Striping tape

Striping brush

Polish palette

POLISH COLOURS

White   Lavender   Blue   Pink

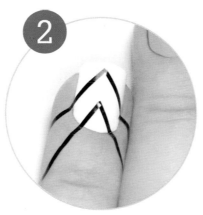

Polish your nails lavender with a white accent nail on your ring finger. Let them dry completely before continuing.

Apply striping tape to the white nail in upwards 'V' shapes, as shown.

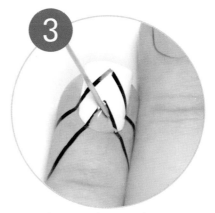

Paint the triangle near the cuticle with lavender polish using your striping brush.

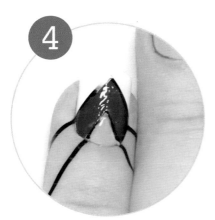

Paint the V-shape in the middle of the nail with blue polish using your striping brush.

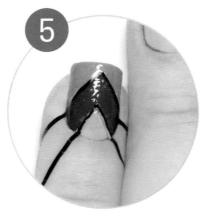

Paint the remaining space near the free edge with pink polish using your striping brush.

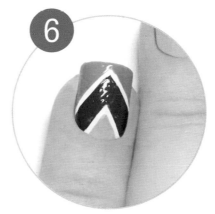

Immediately after polishing, carefully remove the striping tape.

Abstract Roses

Simple brush strokes and dots come together to make graphic, abstract rose motifs in this manicure. Create several roses in different colours on each nail as shown here, or paint one large rose radiating across the entire nail.

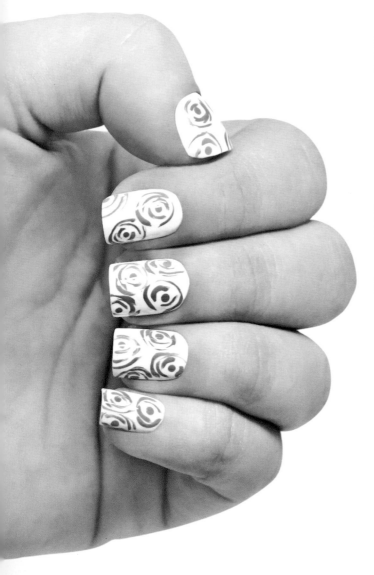

MATERIALS

Dotting tool

Polish palette

Striping brush

POLISH COLOURS

White   Orange   Pink

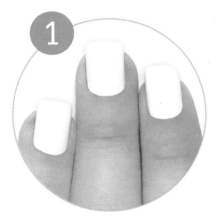

Polish your nails white. Let them dry for a few minutes.

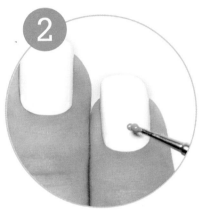

Make a small orange dot on one nail using your dotting tool.

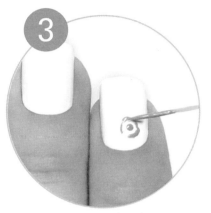

Using your striping brush, create two round shapes encircling the dot in orange polish.

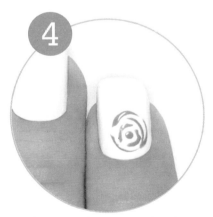

Make several more circular shapes to create a rose.

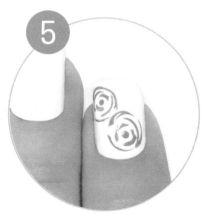

Repeat steps 2 through 4 on the same nail using pink polish.

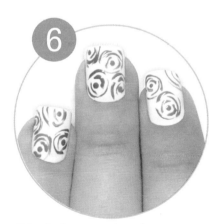

Fill all of your nails with orange and pink roses.

Whimsical Floral

If you aren't yet confident with detailed free-hand work, try this whimsical floral design. Use bright, contrasting shades on a neutral background for an impressive look that is perfect for spring or summer.

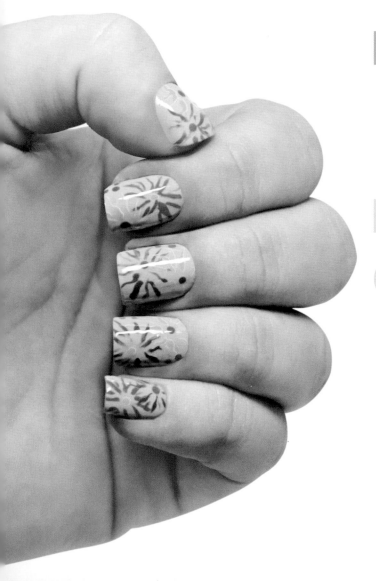

POLISH COLOURS

Beige   Teal   Pink   Purple

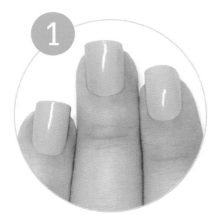

Polish your nails beige. Let them dry for a few minutes.

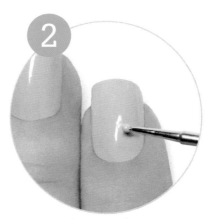

Use your dotting tool to create a small teal dot on one nail.

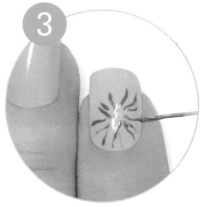

Using your striping brush and pink polish, paint several wiggly lines radiating from the teal dot to resemble long flower petals.

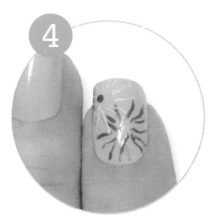

Repeat steps 2 and 3, this time with a purple centre and wiggly lines in teal. The flower petals can overlap.

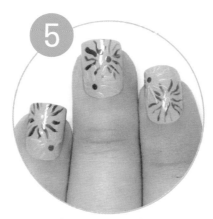

Fill all of your nails with flowers, changing the colour combinations as you go along.

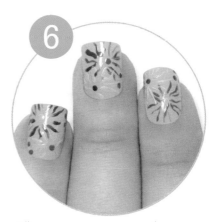

Fill any empty space on the nails with purple, teal, and pink dots.

Sidewall Moons

This monochromatic take on the popular moon manicure features several shades and finishes of pink. For an edgier look, try this manicure in contrasting bold shades.

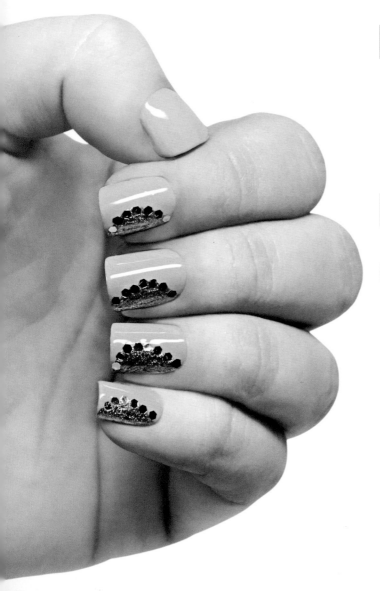

MATERIALS

Striping brush

Polish palette

Top coat (not quick-dry)

Dotting tool

Pink glitter sequins

POLISH COLOURS

Pink

Metallic pink

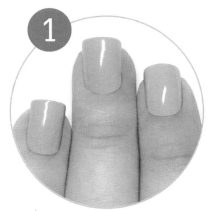

Polish your nails in a pink polish.
Let them dry for a few minutes.

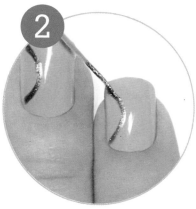

Using your striping brush, create
a curved line near the sidewall
of each nail in metallic pink polish.

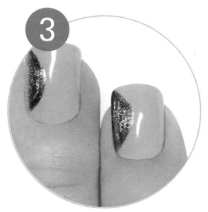

Fill the half-moon shape using
your striping brush and metallic
pink polish.

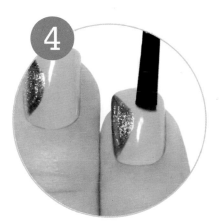

Apply a layer of top coat
to one nail.

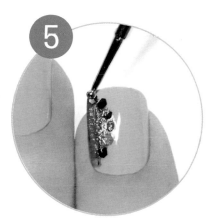

Using a dotting tool dipped in
top coat, place individual pink
glitter sequins along the border
of the half-moon shape.

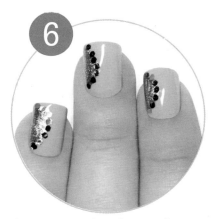

Repeat steps 4 and 5 on all
nails. Seal the glitter sequins in
place with two layers of top coat.

Dot Gradient

The Dot Gradient manicure combines a simple dotting technique with potentially countless colour combinations. Adapt this manicure for different seasons by choosing appropriate colours for your dots. Bold purple and blue dots are great for any time of year.

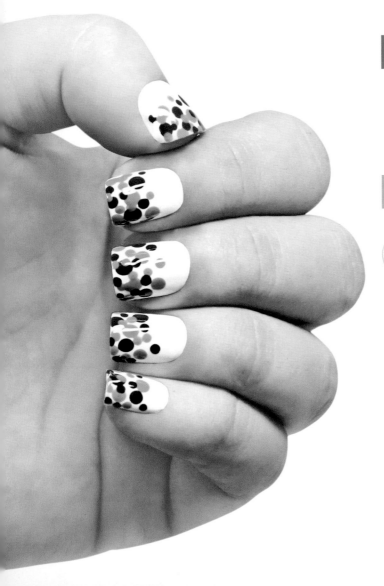

MATERIALS

Dotting tool

Polish palette

POLISH COLOURS

White   Blue   Purple

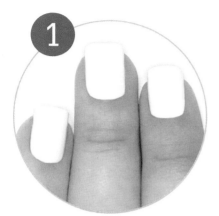

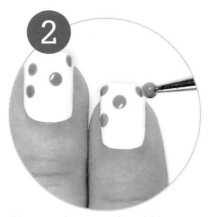

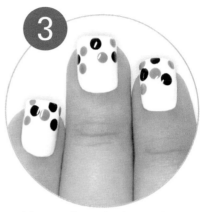

Polish your nails white. Let them dry for a few minutes.

Using a dotting tool and blue polish, paint several large dots on the half of the nail closest to the free edge, but leave some space between the dots.

Add several purple dots to the same area. They can overlap the blue dots.

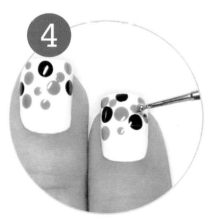

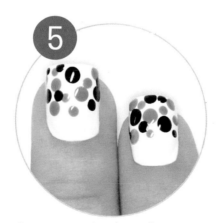

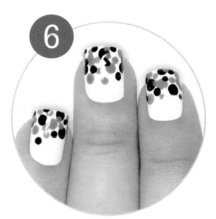

Using the small end of your dotting tool, add small blue dots that overlap the other dots.

Repeat step 4 with small purple dots.

Add more dots to fill in the nail closest to the free edge, producing a gradient effect.

Palm Trees

Heading off to the tropics on holiday? This manicure would be perfect. Or simply use it any time you need to achieve a beach state of mind. The gradient and palm tree silhouettes evoke images of sunsets over the warm ocean.

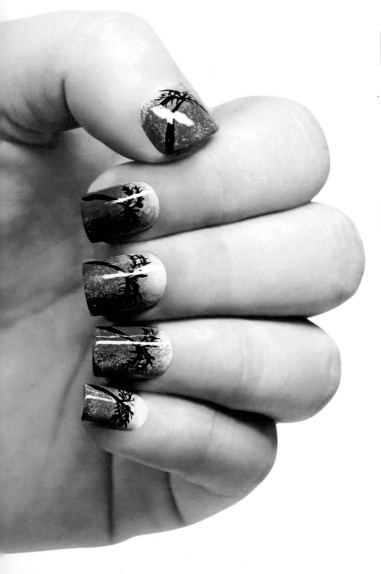

POLISH COLOURS

White   Yellow   Pink   Purple   Black

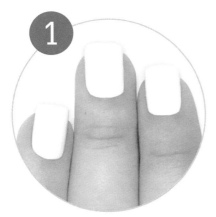

Polish your nails white. Let them dry completely.

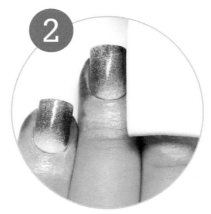

Paint stripes of yellow, pink, and purple polish on a cosmetic sponge and press it on to each nail.

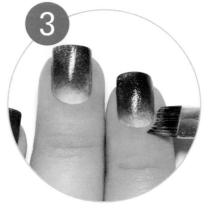

Repeat step 2 until the gradient is vibrant. Remove any excess polish with acetone and angled eyeliner brush.

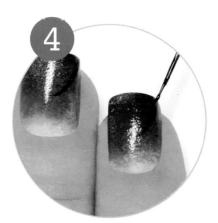

Using your black striping brush and black polish or acrylic paint, paint a curved line from the centre of your nail to one corner of the free edge.

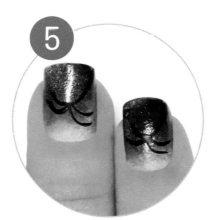

Use your striping brush to create the branches of the palm tree.

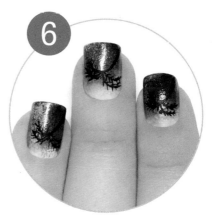

Add short thin lines extending off of each branch until the palm tree is complete. Seal the design with a layer of top coat.

Spring Flowers

These bright spring flowers play on the effect of contrasting black and white with a splash of colour. Use flowing strokes of your striping brush to create artistic flowers all over your nails. For a bolder look, use a range of colours to make the splashes.

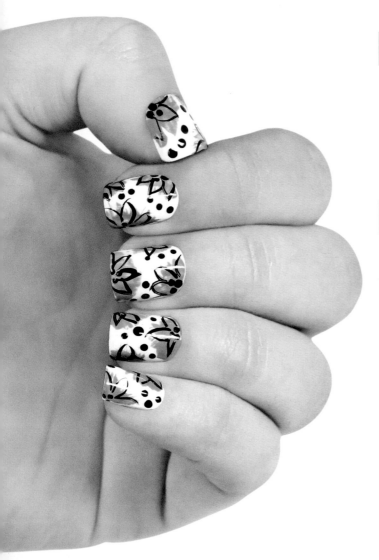

MATERIALS

Striping brush

Polish palette

Dotting tool

POLISH COLOURS

White   Pink   Black

1

Polish your nails with a white polish. Let them dry for a few minutes.

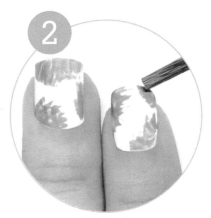

2

Use your polish brush to paint messy pink splashes of colour all over your nails. For a complete look, create some partial splashes at the edges of your nails.

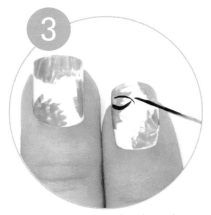

3

Using your striping brush and black polish or acrylic paint, create a petal shape on top of one of the pink splashes.

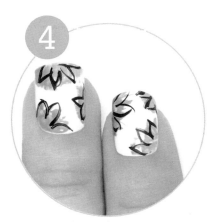

4

Use a similar technique to create flowers with four or five petals on top of each splash.

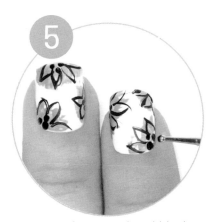

5

Use your dotting tool and black polish to add two or three dots to the centre of each flower.

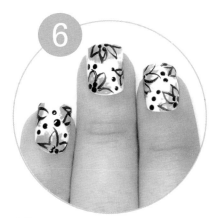

6

Fill any empty space on your nail with black dots.

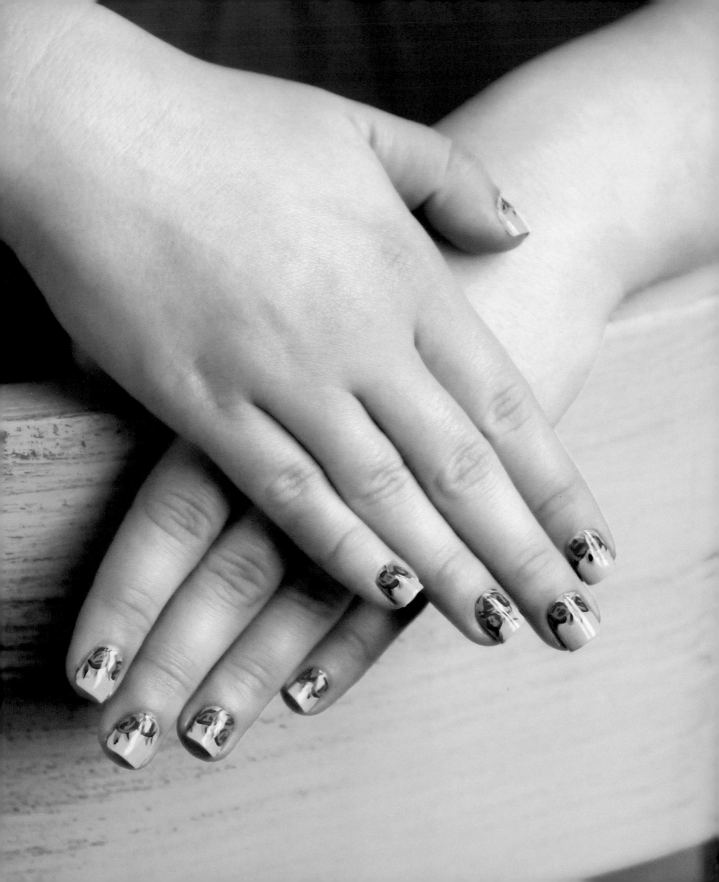

Advanced
Designs

The advanced manicures in this section feature beautiful freehand designs, as well as more complex applications of the basic techniques you have learnt so far. Many of these tutorials require some artistic interpretation, so have fun and express yourself with confidence. As with the previous tutorials in this book, these manicures can be adapted to suit the occasion with different polish shades and finishes.

Zigzags

Zigzag manicures in sharply contrasting shades can look extremely bold, or can be more understated using softer feminine colours. Start with a well spaced grid, so your zigzags will spread evenly across your nails.

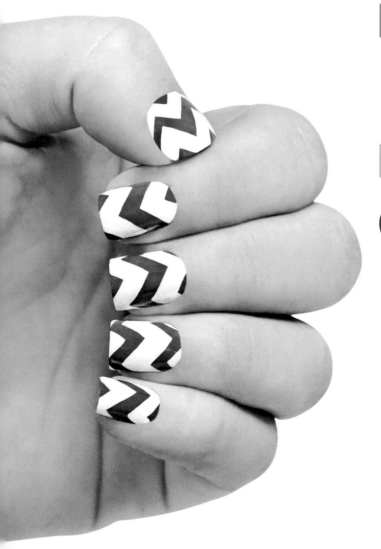

MATERIALS

Striping brush

Polish palette

POLISH COLOURS

Blue   White

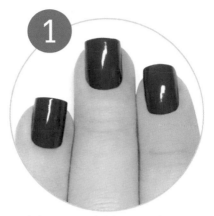

Polish your nails blue. Let them dry for a few minutes.

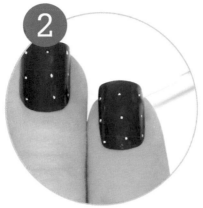

Use the tip of your striping brush and white polish to make a grid of tiny dots across your nails.

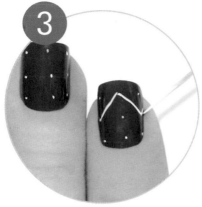

Using your striping brush and white polish or acrylic paint, connect the dots in a zigzag pattern.

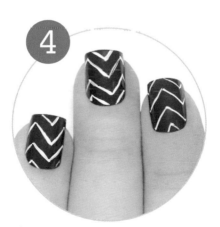

Continue to paint zigzags on your nails until all of the dots of the grids are connected.

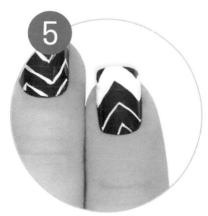

Use your striping brush and white polish to fill in the space between two of the zigzag lines.

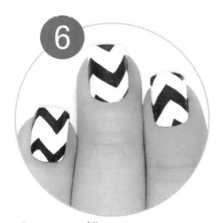

Continue to fill in zigzags, alternating white and blue.

Water Marble

The water marble technique may seem a bit daunting, but the finished look is well worth the time and patience needed. Endless colour combinations and designs can be created and, as with most things, practice makes perfect.

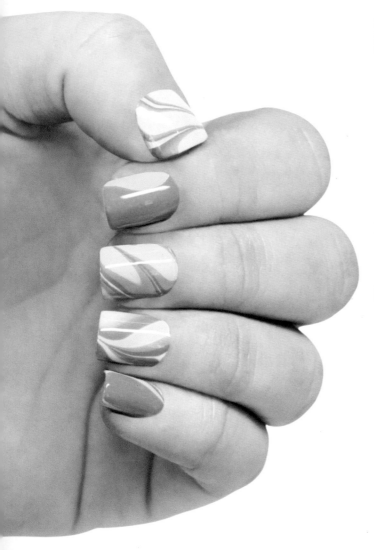

MATERIALS

Kitchen paper	Wooden cocktail sticks
Small cup	Acetone
Water	Clean-up brush
Clear adhesive tape	

POLISH COLOURS

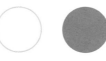

| White | Pink | Grey | Blue |

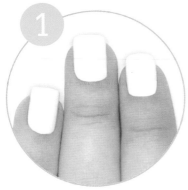

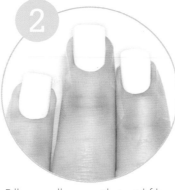

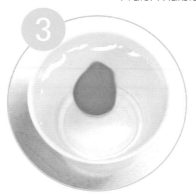

1. Prepare your work area by laying down kitchen paper, if needed. Paint your nails white. Let dry completely.

2. Fill a small cup with tepid filtered or bottled water. Apply clear adhesive tape around your nails to reduce clean-up later.

3. Holding the polish brush over the cup, let a drop of pink polish fall onto the surface of the water and spread out.

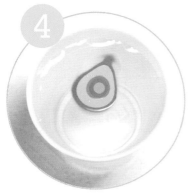

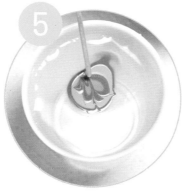

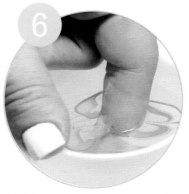

4. Carefully place three to four more drops of polish on top of the first drop. Let each colour spread out before adding the next drop.

5. Drag the tip of a cocktail stick through the polish on the surface of the water, creating the desired design or swirls.

6. Hold your nail is parallel to the water surface. Carefully dip one nail through the polish. Hold it under water until the polish dries.

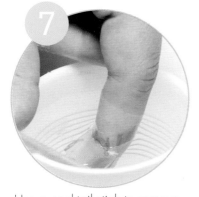

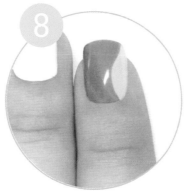

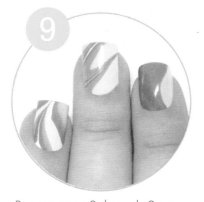

7. Use a cocktail stick to remove the excess dried polish from your skin at the surface of the water.

8. Carefully lift your finger out of the water. Remove the tape and use acetone and the brush to clean up.

9. Repeat steps 3 through 8 on the rest of your nails, or wear a water marble as an accent nail.

Plaid

While the plaid manicure appears to be complex, it is actually just a case of layering simple straight lines. Just take it one step at a time. Try this festive red and green colour scheme, or use one of your own favourite combinations.

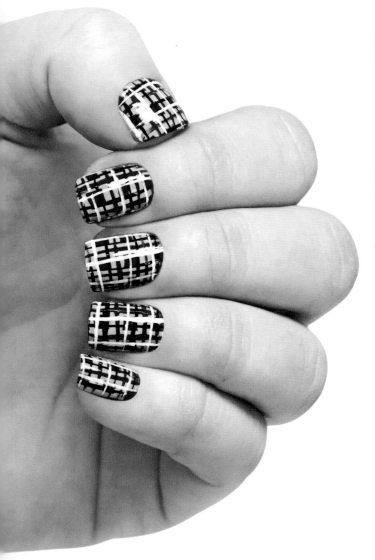

MATERIALS

Striping brush

Polish palette

POLISH COLOURS

| Red | Green | Black | White |

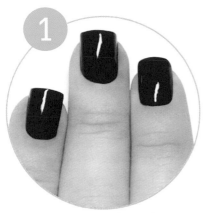

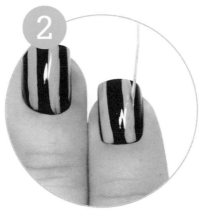

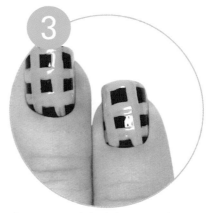

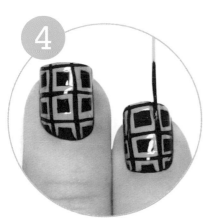

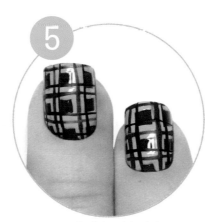

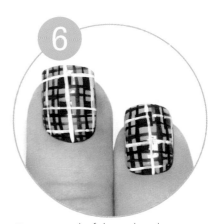

Polish your nails red. Let them dry for a few minutes.

Using your striping brush and green polish, paint several thick vertical lines on to your nails.

Paint several thick horizontal green stripes, creating a series of red squares across your nails.

Use your striping brush and red polish to paint thin lines on top of the thick green ones.

Paint a grid of thin black lines, slightly to the right and above the red lines.

Paint a grid of thin white lines, slightly to the right and above the black ones. Finish the look with a layer of top coat.

Galaxy

The Galaxy manicure uses a simple technique that puts the cosmos at your fingertips. By layering colours with a sponge and adding lots of sparkle, you can create a whole universe of designs.

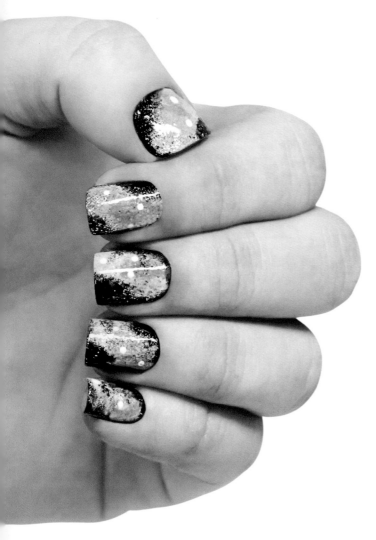

POLISH COLOURS

Black   White   Blue   Green   Purple

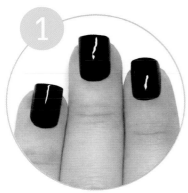

Polish your nails black. Let them dry for a few minutes.

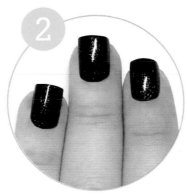

Apply a shimmer top coat over the black polish and let it dry completely.

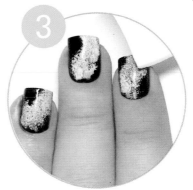

Use a cosmetic sponge to apply a textured band of white polish across each nail. Do not cover the whole nail.

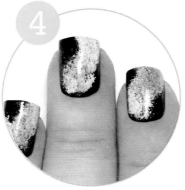

Use a cosmetic sponge to apply some blue polish over the white areas.

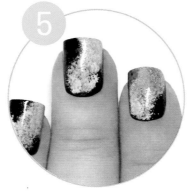

Repeat step 4 with green polish, filling in more of the white space.

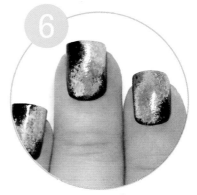

Fill the remainder of the white space by sponging purple polish onto the nails.

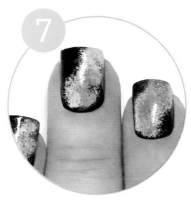

If needed, sponge some black polish around the colours you added to define the galaxies.

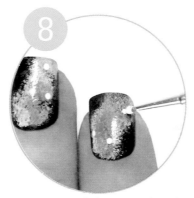

Using a small dotting tool and white polish, apply a few 'stars' to your nails. Let your nails dry.

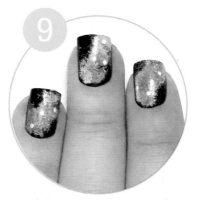

Finish by sponging your nails with fine glitter polish to add a subtle amount of sparkle.

Beach Waves

This abstract manicure is reminiscent of a bird's-eye view of ocean waves hitting a sandy shore. Be imaginative when you apply the strokes of polish to create a flowing gradient of blues and teals, complete with breaking waves at the coastline.

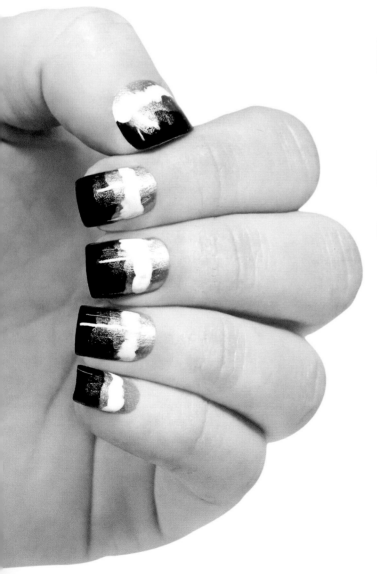

MATERIALS

Top coat

POLISH COLOURS

Gold   Navy blue   Blue metallic   Teal   White

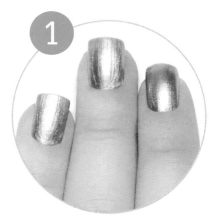

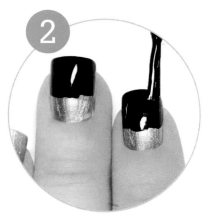

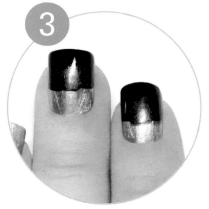

Paint your nails gold. Let them dry for a few minutes.

Using the brush from the bottle, apply a thin coat of navy polish from halfway down the nail to the free edge.

Paint over the lower half of the navy section in blue metallic polish. Use irregular strokes to create the look of shallower water close to the gold 'sand'.

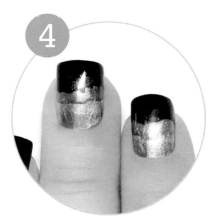

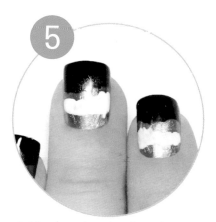

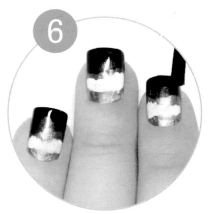

Using the same technique, apply a layer of teal polish overlapping the blue and covering some of the gold.

Add a few short brush strokes of white polish where the blue and gold colours meet to represent the breaking waves.

Apply a top coat to blend the colours together slightly and complete the look.

Angular Moons

This manicure requires an extremely steady hand, but the final result is well worth the time and focus demanded. For detailed work like this, acrylic paint works best as it dries quickly and stays exactly where you apply it.

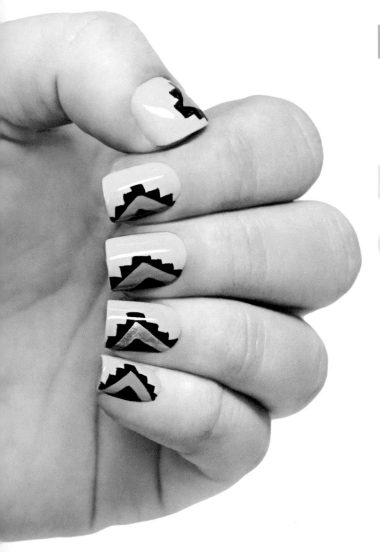

MATERIALS

Striping brush

Polish palette

POLISH COLOURS

| Beige | Black | Blue | Gold |

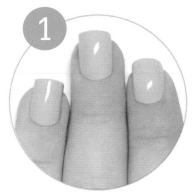

Paint your nails beige. Let them dry for a few minutes.

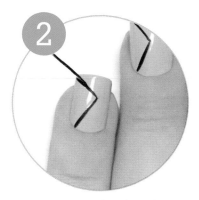

Using a striping brush and black polish or acrylic paint, make a V-shape coming from the sidewall of each nail.

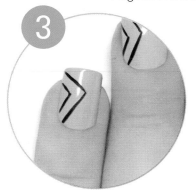

Paint a second V-shape within the first one, closer to the sidewall.

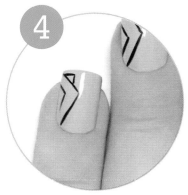

Carefully paint a small right angle coming off the V-shape you made in step 2.

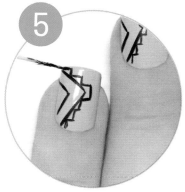

Repeat step 4, adding right angles round the entire V-shape on all of your nails.

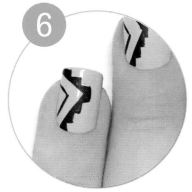

Carefully use your striping brush to fill in the angles with black polish or acrylic paint.

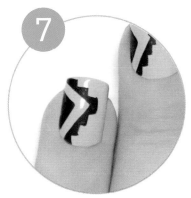

Fill the space between the sidewall and smallest V-shape with black polish or acrylic paint.

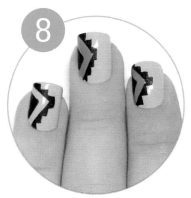

On all of your nails except your ring finger nail, fill in the final V-shape with blue polish.

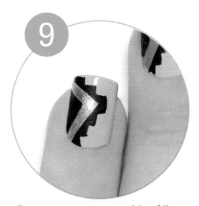

Create an accent nail by filling the final V-shape on your ring finger nail with gold polish.

Sugar Skulls

This tutorial combines several techniques to create a quirky sugar skull. Whether you decide to wear this nail art as an accent nail or sport ten little skulls, this manicure is sure to attract attention.

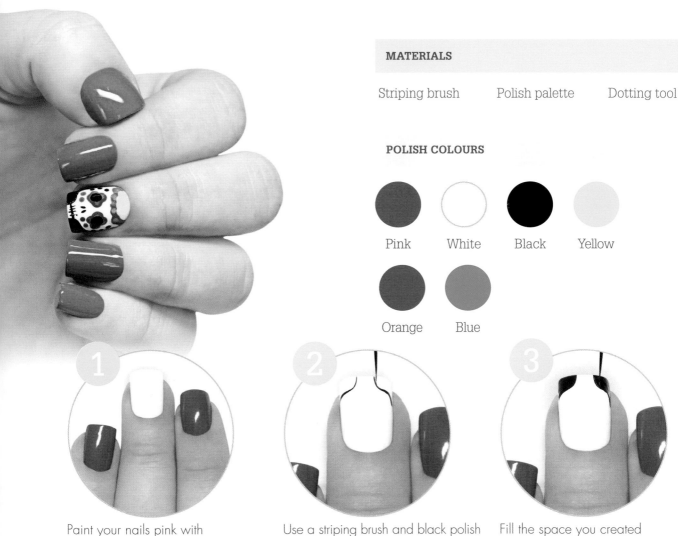

MATERIALS

Striping brush   Polish palette   Dotting tool

POLISH COLOURS

Pink   White   Black   Yellow

Orange   Blue

1
Paint your nails pink with one white accent nail. Let them dry for a few minutes.

2
Use a striping brush and black polish to draw a jawline using two curved lines on the accent nail, from the sidewall to the free edge.

3
Fill the space you created in step 2 with black polish.

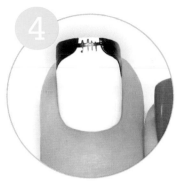

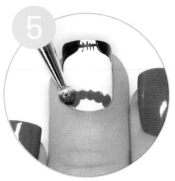

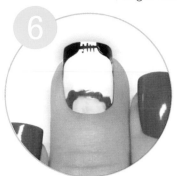

Use your striping brush and black polish to paint the lip line with teeth along it, creating a mouth.

Use a dotting tool and pink polish to create a semi-circle of overlapping dots near the base of the nail.

Use your dotting tool to fill the space between the pink dots and the base of the nail with yellow polish.

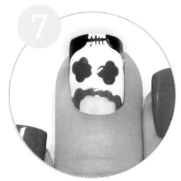

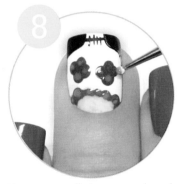

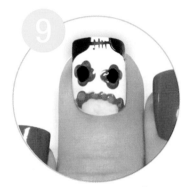

Use your dotting tool and orange polish to create two sets of four overlapping dots in a cross shape.

Using a small dotting tool and blue polish, add small accent dots to the pink and orange dots.

Add the eye sockets to the skulls with black polish and a dotting tool.

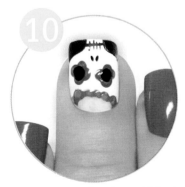

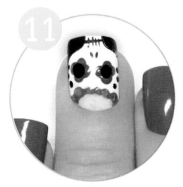

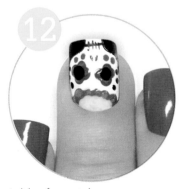

Use a striping brush and black polish to paint two angled lines, creating a nose.

Using a small dotting tool and black polish, add a few accent dots on the outside of the eyes.

Add a few pink accent dots where the cheekbones would be.

Ice Cream Cones

For a guilt-free treat, why not enjoy some luxurious ice cream on your nails? Play with different polish colours for your ice cream tips to mimic your favourite flavours. The ice cream in this tutorial is mint chocolate chip.

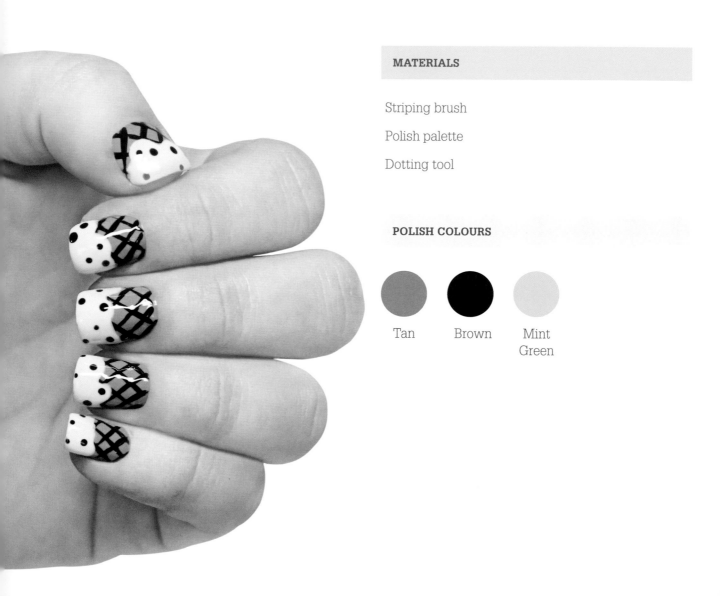

MATERIALS

Striping brush

Polish palette

Dotting tool

POLISH COLOURS

Tan   Brown   Mint Green

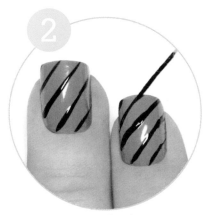

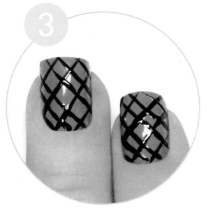

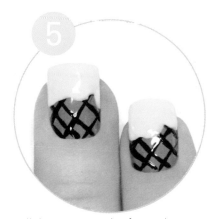

Polish your nails in tan polish. Let them dry for a few minutes.

Use your striping brush to paint a series of brown diagonal lines across your nails.

Paint a series of lines crossing the ones you painted in step 2, creating a grid.

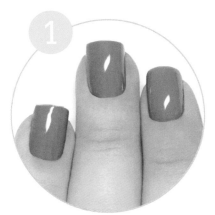

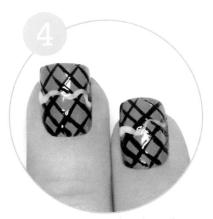

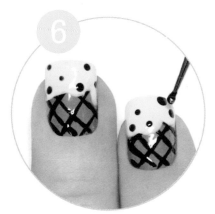

Using your striping brush and mint green polish, paint a crooked line near your free edge.

Fill the space at the free edge using your striping brush and the mint green polish.

Add a few brown dots on the mint green polish. These are chocolate chips.

Jack-o'-Lantern

You can't go wrong with jack-o'-lantern nails for Hallowe'en. This tutorial shows you how to create a traditional jack-o'-lantern accent nail, but feel free to use your own ideas when painting the shape of the eyes, nose, and mouth.

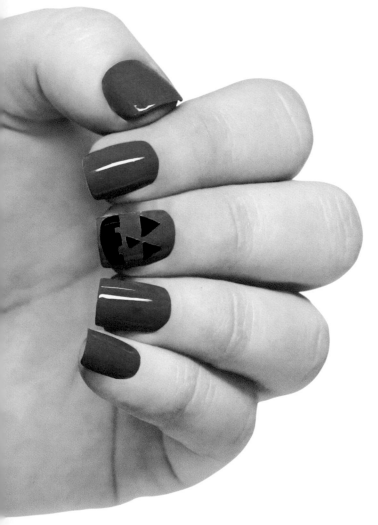

MATERIALS

Striping brush

Polish palette

POLISH COLOURS

Orange   Black

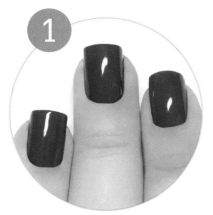

Polish your nails orange. Let them dry for a few minutes.

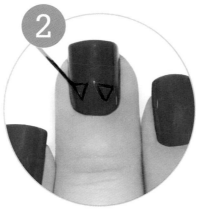

Use your striping brush and black polish or acrylic paint to create two small triangles. These are the jack-o'-lantern's eyes.

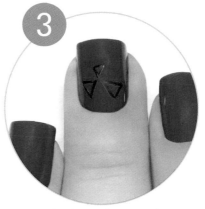

Paint a third, smaller triangle centred on the nail. This is the jack-o'-lantern's nose.

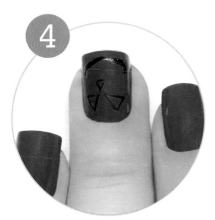

Create the beginning of the mouth by painting a curved line near your free edge.

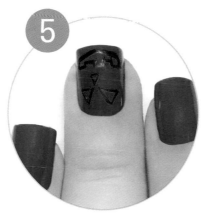

Finish the mouth with a notched line across the top.

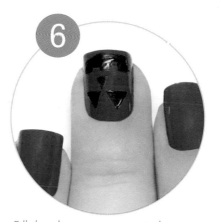

Fill the shapes you created in the previous steps with black polish or acrylic paint.

Tartan

This variation on a plaid manicure is perfectly sophisticated and would be brilliant for the festive season. Once you have mastered basic stripes, this manicure will be well within your skill set.

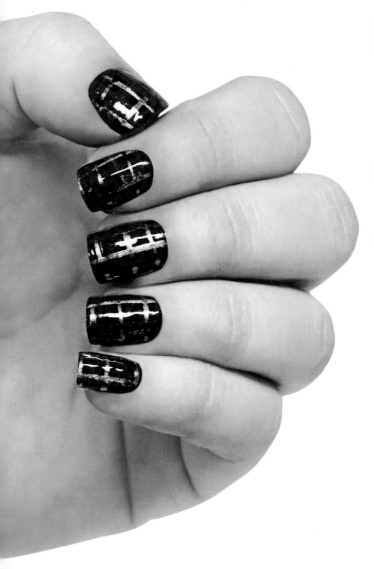

MATERIALS

Striping brush

Polish palette

POLISH COLOURS

| Navy | Red | Red Metallic | Dark Green | Gold |

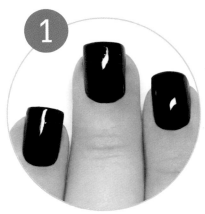

Polish your nails navy blue. Let them dry for a few minutes.

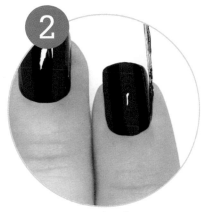

Using a striping brush, paint thick vertical stripes in a red polish. Evenly space them across your nail.

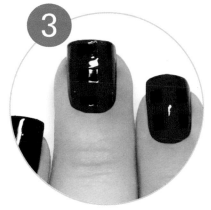

Using the same method, create thick red horizontal stripes that overlap the vertical ones.

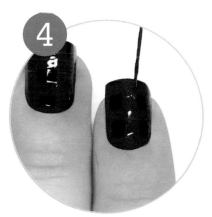

Where the red stripes overlap, paint metallic red squares with your striping brush to add shimmer to the design.

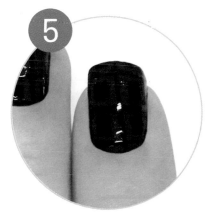

Again using a striping brush, paint thin dark green stripes centred over the thick red stripes.

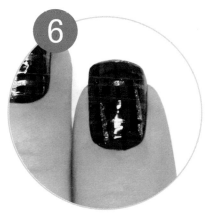

Paint thin gold stripes centred over the space between the red stripes.

Safari Nails

This manicure combines three sensational nail art techniques: sponging, leopard, and zebra. They come together to produce a playfully wild design. This tutorial features bright shades, but you could use earth tones for a more natural look.

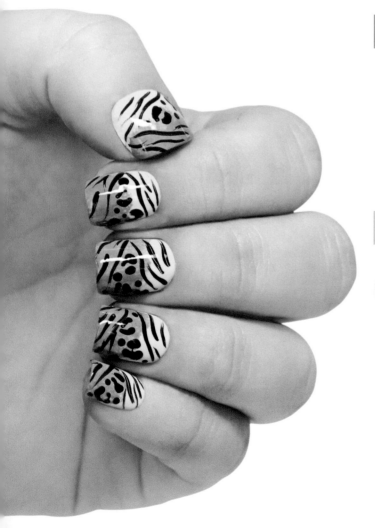

POLISH COLOURS

Yellow   Pink   Black

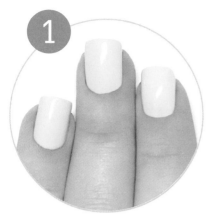

Polish your nails in yellow polish. Let them dry for a few minutes.

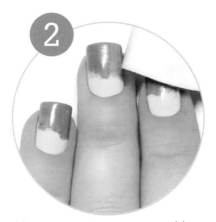

Use a cosmetic sponge to add some pink polish to the tips of your nails. This does not need to be perfect.

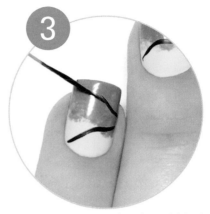

Using your striping brush and black polish or acrylic paint, make two slightly wiggly lines coming to a point near the sidewall.

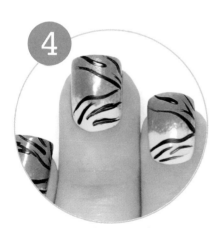

Create several more zebra stripes, filling the spaces near the free edge and the base of the nail.

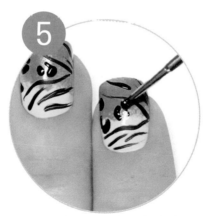

Use your dotting tool and black polish to create small leopard spots in the remaining space. C-shapes work well.

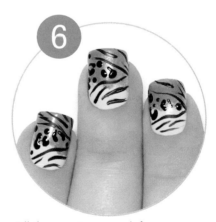

Fill the empty space left on your nails with small black dots.

Jingle Bells

This manicure is just perfect for the festive season. The contrast between metallic and crème polishes and the detail on the bells make for a celebratory design that can be used on all ten nails or as an accent nail.

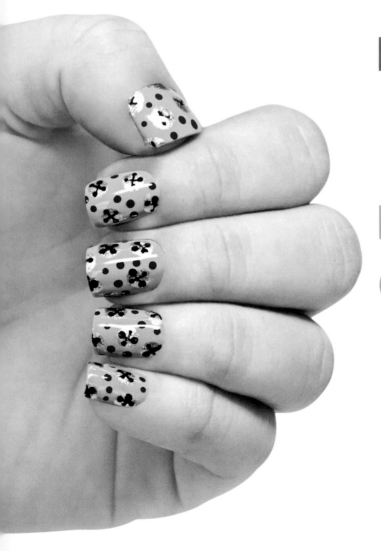

POLISH COLOURS

Green   Gold   Silver   Black   Red

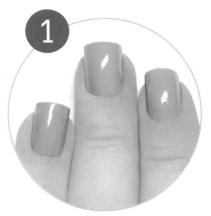

Polish your nails green. Let them dry for a few minutes.

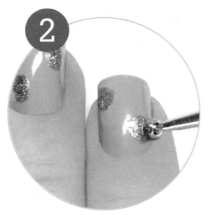

Use your dotting tool and gold polish to make several large dots. Spread them out across your nails.

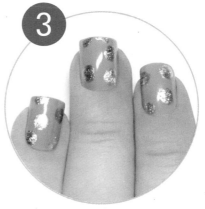

Use the same technique to create several large silver dots.

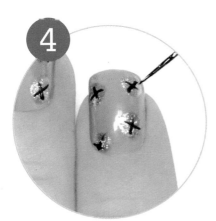

Use your striping brush and black polish or acrylic paint to make a small '+' shape on each circle.

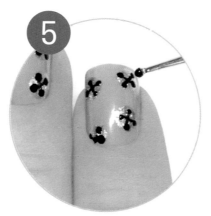

Use the small end of your dotting tool and black polish to add tiny dots to the ends of each '+' sign.

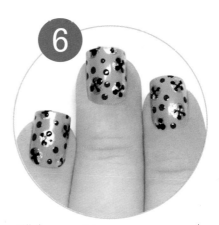

Fill the remaining spaces on each nail with small red dots.

Candy Canes

Striping tape and festive polish colours come together in this Christmas manicure. You could use your striping brush to paint these stripes, but the tape creates crisp lines in red and green to emulate a traditional Christmas treat.

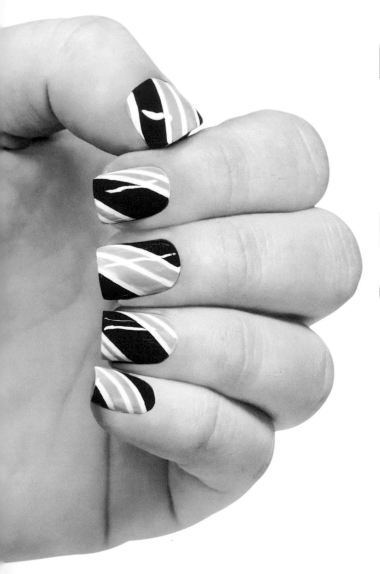

Striping tape

Striping brush

Polish palette

POLISH COLOURS

White   Red   Green

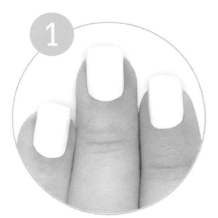

Paint your nails white.
Let them dry completely.

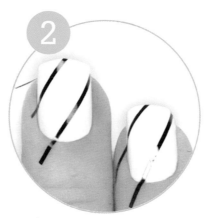

Apply striping tape to your
nails on the diagonal, spread
widely across the nail plate.

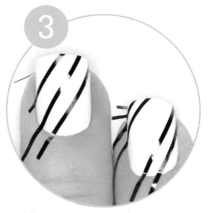

Add another piece of striping
tape between the pieces you
placed in step 2. Do this
between every other piece.

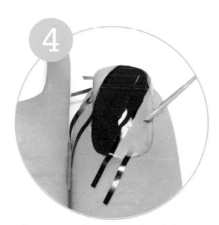

On one nail, paint red polish
over the widely spaced tape
and green over the sections
with two pieces of tape.

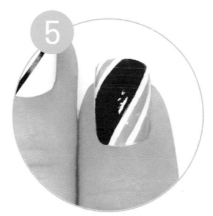

Immediately after polishing,
carefully remove the tape.

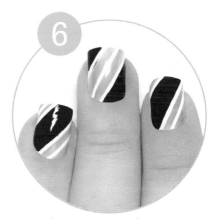

Complete steps 4 and 5
on the rest of your nails,
one nail at a time.

Fairy Lights

This decorative manicure uses strokes of your striping brush to represent a string of coloured fairy lights dancing across your nails. You could use this design on its own or as one element in a manicure combined with several others for the festive season.

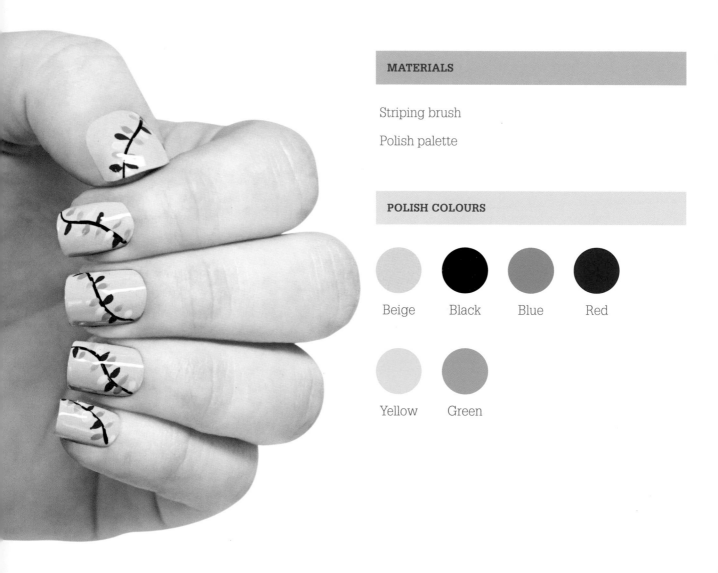

MATERIALS

Striping brush

Polish palette

POLISH COLOURS

Beige   Black   Blue   Red

Yellow   Green

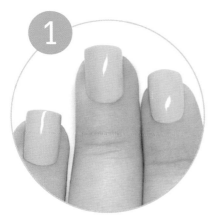

Paint your nails beige. Let them dry for a few minutes.

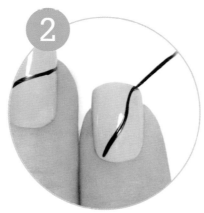

Use your striping brush and black polish or acrylic paint to create a curved line across each nail.

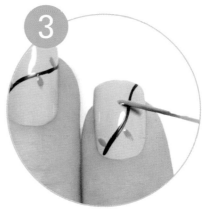

Use your striping brush to add tiny fairy lights along the black line in blue polish.

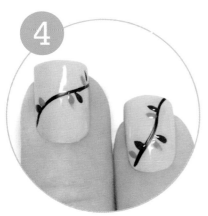

Using a similar technique, add red fairy lights.

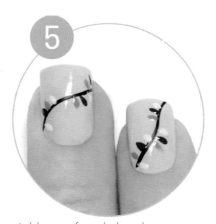

Add more fairy lights, this time in yellow polish.

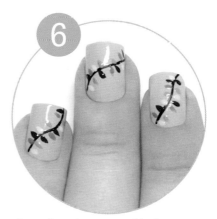

Complete the string of lights with green bulbs, and fill any remaining spaces with colours of your choice.

Detailed Roses

There are few nail art designs more feminine than those using roses, and soft details along with multiple shades of pink and green bring the blooms to life on your nails. The bold teal base colour pops against the pinks of the flowers.

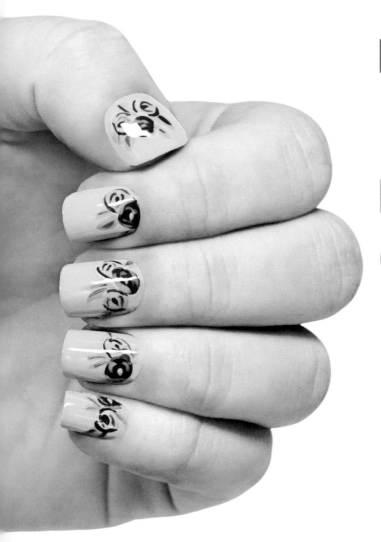

MATERIALS

Striping brush

Polish palette

POLISH COLOURS

| Teal | Light pink | Dark pink | Light green | Dark green |

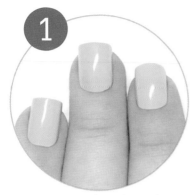

Polish your nails teal. Let them dry for a few minutes.

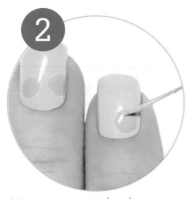

Use your striping brush to paint one or two circular shapes in light pink polish near the base of each nail.

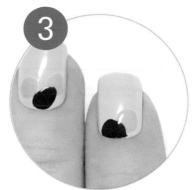

Add a dark pink circular shape to each nail, creating clusters of roses.

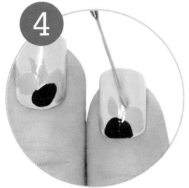

Use your striping brush and light green polish to paint several triangular leaves on each cluster of roses.

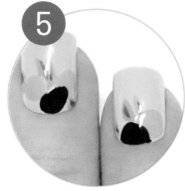

Use your striping brush and dark green polish to add a short detail line down the centre of each leaf.

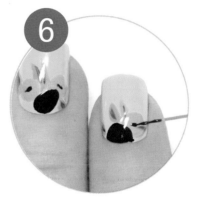

Use your striping brush and dark pink polish to add a small dot mark at the centre of each light pink rose.

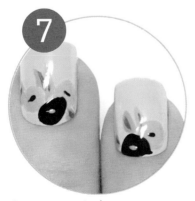

Repeat step 6, this time placing light pink dot marks in each dark pink rose.

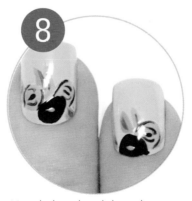

Use dark pink polish and your striping brush to add subtle detail to the light pink roses. Round shapes work well.

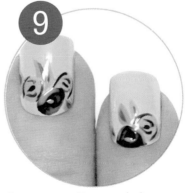

Repeat step 8, using light pink polish to add detail to the dark pink roses.

Crisscross

This graphic manicure brings together short line segments to create an eye-catching design. The neon pink polish used here is perfect for the summer, but you could change the colour scheme of this design to fit any season or occasion.

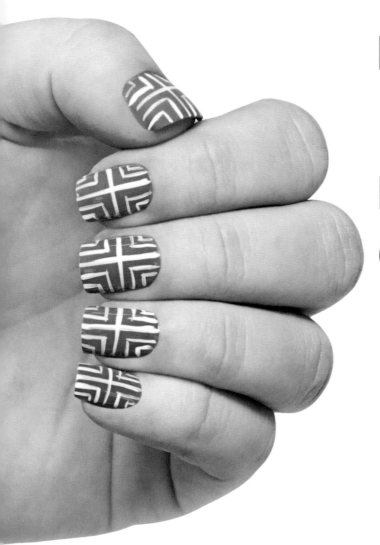

MATERIALS

Striping brush

Polish palette

POLISH COLOURS

Neon pink

White

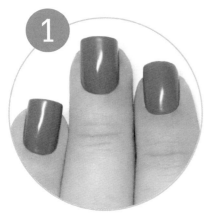

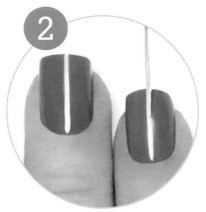

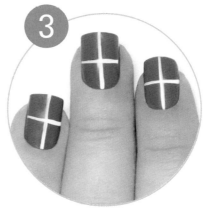

Paint your nails neon pink. Let them dry for a few minutes.

Use your striping brush and white polish or acrylic paint to make a vertical line down the centre of each nail.

Paint a white horizontal line on each nail, creating a cross shape.

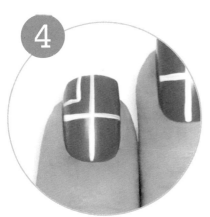

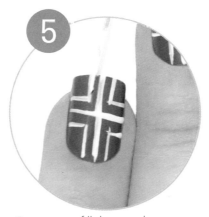

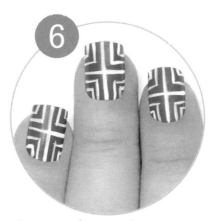

In one of the quadrants created by the cross, paint two small line segments, following the shape of the original lines.

Continue to fill the quadrants of the manicure with line segments using white polish or acrylic paint.

If the size of your nails permits, add another set of lines to each nail.

Fire Manicure

Flames on your nails make a feisty statement. This tutorial explains
how to do a fiery red flame, but you could also put together a
scheme using cooler colours to create a unique gradient look.

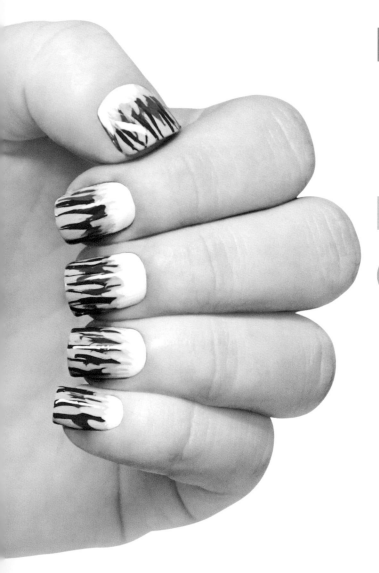

MATERIALS

Striping brush

Polish palette

Top coat

POLISH COLOURS

Grey   Red   Orange   Yellow   White

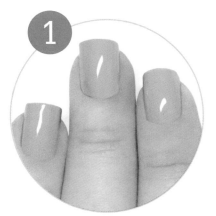

Paint your nails grey. Let them dry for a few minutes.

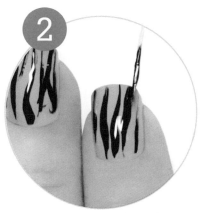

Use your striping brush and red polish to create a series of brushstrokes across most of the nail.

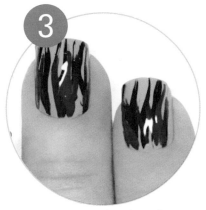

Use your striping brush and orange polish to add orange brushstrokes, leaving some red exposed near the free edge.

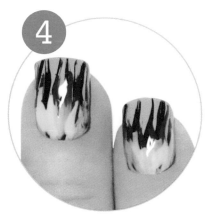

Using a similar technique, apply some yellow brushstrokes to your nail, closer to the base.

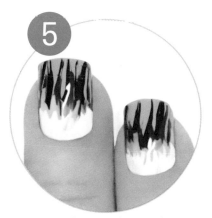

Finish the 'fire' gradient with some short white brushstrokes at the very base of your nail.

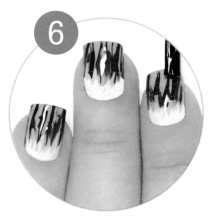

Apply a top coat to smooth the colours of the fire gradient.

Union Jack

Flags tend to be colourful and graphic in design. With its sharp angles and contrasting colours, the Union Jack is a famous example. Wear this design as an accent nail with a classy red manicure.

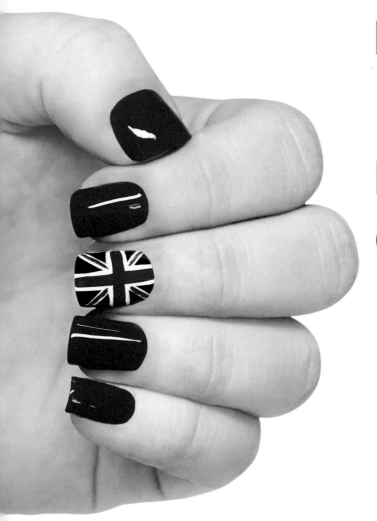

MATERIALS

Striping brush

Polish palette

POLISH COLOURS

Blue   Red   White

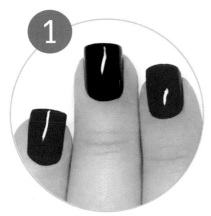

Polish your nails red with a blue accent nail. Let them dry for a few minutes.

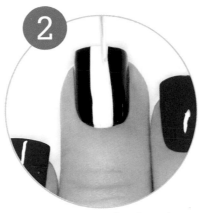

Using your striping brush and white polish, paint a thick white line vertically down the centre of your accent nail.

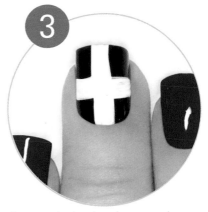

Paint a thick white horizontal line across the centre of your nail, creating a cross shape.

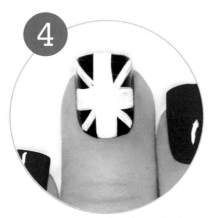

Use your striping brush and white polish to paint an X-shape over the cross. These lines should be slightly thinner.

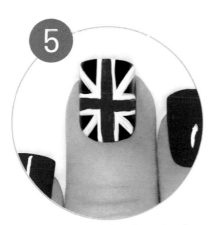

Use your striping brush and red polish to paint a red cross layered over the white one. Leave a white border on either side of the lines.

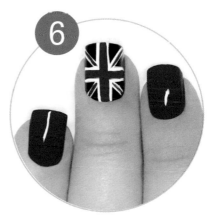

Finish with thin red lines layered over the white X-shape. Leave a white border on either side and between the red X-shape and the cross.

Bull's-eye Dots

This manicure is made up of layered dots that create a bull's-eye pattern. Take your time to let the dots dry so the polish does not get too thick. As always, be imaginative with your colour choices; the possibilities are endless.

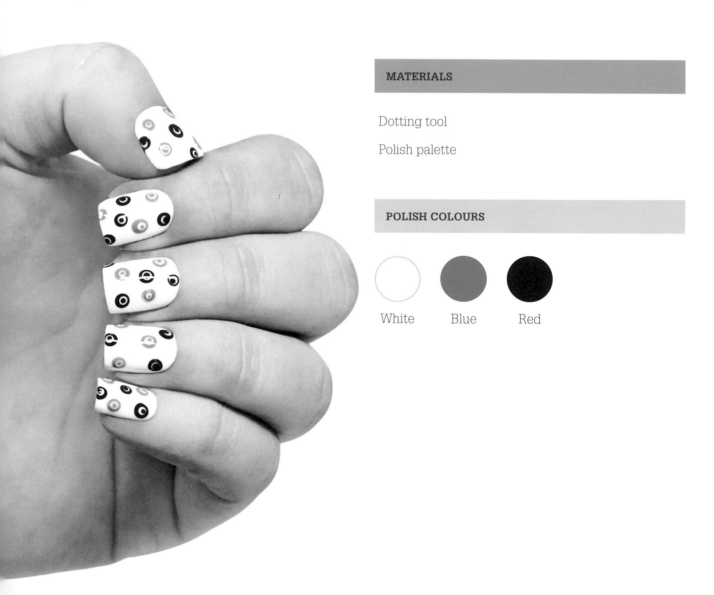

MATERIALS

Dotting tool

Polish palette

POLISH COLOURS

White   Blue   Red

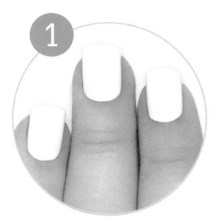

Paint your nails white. Let them dry for a few minutes.

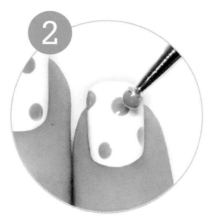

Use your dotting tool to create blue dots, placed randomly across your nails.

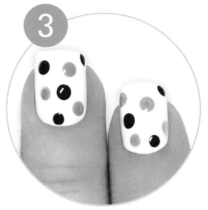

Use your dotting tool and red polish to add some red dots, placed randomly on the nails.

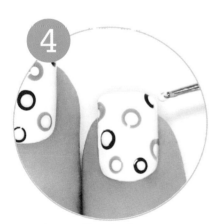

Use the small end of your dotting tool to place white dots in the centre of all of the red and blue dots.

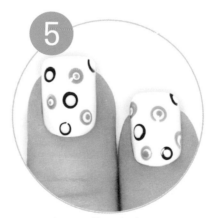

Using the small end of your dotting tool, carefully apply tiny blue dots to the centre of the blue dots with white centres.

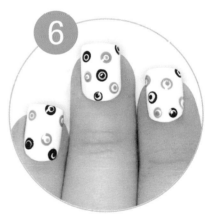

Repeat step 5, this time with red polish on the red dots with white centres.

Glossary

2-FREE Term used to describe a top coat formula made with DBP or toluene, but that does not contain formaldehyde or dibutyl phthalate.

3-FREE Term used to describe a product that does not include formaldehyde, toluene, or dibutyl phthalate.

ACCENT NAIL One or two nails polished differently to the other nails in a manicure.

ACETONE Strong solvent used to remove nail polish and soak-off gel manicures.

BASE COAT A clear coat applied to the nail to prevent staining and help with polish adhesion.

BIG 3 A group of potentially harmful chemicals including formaldehyde, toluene, and dibutyl phthalate.

BUFFER A high-grit file used to smooth the nail plate.

CAMPHOR A potentially irritating chemical.

CLEAN-UP BRUSH A brush, such as an angled eyeliner brush, used to remove excess polish.

CLEAR ADHESIVE TAPE Regular plastic adhesive tape that can also be used in nail art.

COSMETIC SPONGE A disposable sponge wedge that can be used to apply polish.

CUTICLE see True Cuticle.

CUTICLE NIPPER A manicure tool used to remove dead tissue from the nail plate.

CUTICLE OIL A mixture of moisturizing oils used on the nail and surrounding skin.

CUTICLE PUSHER A manicure tool used to gently scrape dead cuticle tissue from the nail plate.

CUTICLE REMOVER A cream or gel containing chemicals that dissolve dead skin from the nail plate.

DEHYDRATOR A product used to dry the nail plate in preparation for a soak-off gel manicure.

DIBUTYL PHTHALATE (DBP) One of the Big 3 chemicals.

DOTTING TOOL Nail art tool with a round end that creates a dot when pressed to the nail.

EPONYCHIUM Living tissue at the base of the nail plate that creates a seal with the skin.

FILE An abrasive tool used to remove length and shape the free edge of the nail.

FOIL METHOD A method used to remove glitter polish and soak-off gel manicures that involves placing a cotton wool ball soaked in acetone against the nail plate and wrapping the fingertip in foil to seal it.

FOOT FILE An abrasive tool used to smooth rough, dead skin on the feet.

FORMALDEHYDE One of the Big 3 chemicals. With use over time it can eventually cause the nail plate to become brittle.

FREE EDGE The part of the nail that grows beyond the fingertip.

HAND CREAM Moisturizing cream or lotion used on the fingertips and hands.

HYPONYCHIUM Living tissue under the free edge of the nail that creates a seal with the skin.

JOJOBA OIL A natural oil that can penetrate the nail plate.

KERATIN A protein that makes up the hair, skin, and nails.

LANULA The white, moon-shaped part of the nail matrix that is visible under the nail plate.

LATERAL FOLD Living tissue that creates a seal on the sidewall of the nail with the skin.

LED LAMP An electric lamp used to cure soak-off gel manicures.

MANICURE The act of caring for and beautifying the hands and fingernails.

NAIL ADHESIVE Glue used to adhere 3D elements to the nail plate.

NAIL ART TWEEZERS Tweezers with a bent, elongated end used to apply 3D elements to the nail plate.

NAIL CHARM 3D element in any shape that can be applied to the nail plate.

NAIL CLIPPER A manicure tool used to remove length from the free edge of the nail.

NAIL FOIL Metallic foil on a clear backing.

NAIL MATRIX The living portion of the nail where new cells are created.

NAIL PLATE The hard portion of the nail that is polished.

NAIL TREATMENT A clear, brush-on product that contains proteins or chemicals to encourage nail strength and growth.

PEDICURE The art of caring for and beautifying the feet and toenails.

POLISH PALETTE A piece of stiff material, such as a paper plate or aluminium foil, used to hold puddles of polish for nail art.

SCRUB An abrasive cream or gel that exfoliates the hands or feet.

SHEA BUTTER Natural butter with healing and moisturizing qualities.

SIDEWALL The left and right edges of the nails.

SKITTLE MANICURE A manicure in which each nail is painted in a different colour or pattern.

SOAK-OFF GEL A type of nail polish that is cured under a UV or LED lamp and requires soaking in acetone for removal.

STRIPING BRUSH A long thin paint brush used for nail art.

STRIPING TAPE Thin tape that is designed specifically for creating crisp lines in nail art.

STUD A small, flat-backed metallic 3D element that can be attached to the nail plate.

TOLUENE One of the Big 3 chemicals.

TOP COAT A clear, brush-on product that helps protect your manicure and add shine.

TRUE CUTICLE The dead, sticky white tissue that forms on your nail plate.

UV LAMP An electric lamp used to cure soak-off gel manicures.

WHITENING SOAK Soak used to remove stains from the nail plate. It is available in beauty supply shops or can be made at home.

Resources

In this section, you will find resources to help you navigate the world of nail art. There are plenty of websites, blogs, and magazines full of information and inspiration. Also included here is a list of stockists that carry the products used in this book, as well as some of the top brands for nail art and nail care supplies.

WEBSITES Find inspiration from these great websites that feature nail art.

NAIL IT!
(nailitmag.com)

NAILPRO
(nailpro.com)

NAILS MAGAZINE
(nailsmag.com/style/nail-art)

PINTEREST
(pinterest.com/all/hair_beauty/)

BLOGS Stay up-to-date on everything that's new in the world of nail art with these bloggers.

ADVENTURES IN ACETONE
(adventuresinacetone.com)
Nail art and easy step-by-step tutorials

CHALKBOARD NAILS (chalkboardnails.com)
Innovative nail art

CHICKETTES (chickettes.com)
Gel polishes and nail art

COSMETIC SANCTUARY (cosmeticsanctuary.com)
Nail polish reviews

POINTLESS CAFÉ (pointlesscafe.com)
Nail polish reviews and nail art

SMASHLEY SPARKLES (smashleysparkles.com)
The authority on water marbling

THE NAILASAURUS (thenailasaurus.com)
Cardiff-based nail blogger who also lists a set of links to the best British nail bloggers

THE LACQUEROLOGIST (lacquerologist.com)
Nail art by Emily Draher

WONDROUSLY POLISHED (wondrouslypolished.com)
Detailed nail art

STOCKISTS Purchase nail polish and nail art supplies from these online retailers.

AMAZON
(amazon.co.uk)

ETSY
(etsy.com)

SEPHORA
(sephora.com)

BORN PRETTY STORE
(bornprettystore.com)

HEAD2TOE BEAUTY
(head2toebeauty.com)

SPARKLY NAILS
(sparkly-nails.co.uk)

EBAY
(ebay.co.uk)

MASH NAILS
(mashnails.com)

VIVA LA NAILS
(vivalanails.co.uk)

RECOMMENDED PRODUCTS
Achieve the results you want with some of the best nail care brands. Whether
you buy your favourites at a beauty supply shop, professional salon, or online,
there are countless stockists selling all kinds of brands for you to discover.

JACAVA LONDON (available at jacava.com)
High-gloss, long-lasting nail polish free from 9 toxic
ingredients known to cause health problems. Cruelty
free, it has never been tested on animals.

GEL-CURING LAMPS (nailpolishdirect.co.uk)
Professional-quality manicure and pedicure products
and tools, including UV and LED gel-curing lamps. Try
their cuticle removers and natural nail files.

OUT THE DOOR (available at beautyexpress.co.uk)
3-free, super fast-drying American top coat brand.

OPI (sallyexpress.com)
A reliable supplier for stocking up on iconic, salon-quality
nail brands such as OPI, Seche, SPI, and China Glaze
nail polishes, as well as nail art tools.

NAIL ART TOOLS (thenailartcompany.co.uk)
Online polish and nail care suppliers of professional
quality products, materials, and tools. Founded and
operated by an experienced and fully qualified
professional nail technician, the company continually
researches and sources new nail art tools to bring
customers the very latest in trends and designs.

WET N WILD (available from cosmeticsfairy.co.uk)
This highly popular American brand is a cruelty-free
nail polish that has never been tested on animals.

ZOYA NAIL POLISH (available at tnbl.co.uk and
beautyexpress.co.uk) Zoya make long-wearing,
toxin-free nail polishes and treatment formulas
that contain no formaldehyde, formaldehyde
resin, toluene, dibutyl phthalate (DBP), or camphor.

INDEX

ABOUT THE AUTHOR

Emily Draher is a nail art blogger who writes "The Lacquerologist" (lacquerologist.com), which focuses exclusively on nails: nail polish swatches, nail art, nail and cuticle care, tutorials, and reviews. She is a natural nails nail tech, nail artist, and small business owner at Body*Spa*Banquet Nails in Canton, Ohio. Emily set aside her former career as a biologist to focus on the creativity involved in nail art, and on making people feel happy and empowered through beautiful and expressive manicures.

Acknowledgements

Thank you to everyone who understood and supported me on this colourful journey over the past several years. To Benn, who doesn't care that our house smells like nail polish all the time, and Nance who doesn't mind that her daughter isn't a doctor. I owe a huge thanks to Debbie for all of her hard work and patience creating the images in this book. And to all of my clients, family, and friends who have shared in my excitement: I love you all!